WORLD HEALTH ORGANIZATION

INTERNATIONAL AGENCY FOR RESEARCH
ON CANCER

DIET, HORMONES AND CANCER: METHODOLOGICAL ISSUES FOR PROSPECTIVE STUDIES

EDITORS

E. Riboli and R. Saracci

IARC TECHNICAL REPORT No. 4   Lyon, 1988

Published by the International Agency for Research on Cancer
150 cours Albert Thomas, 69372 Lyon Cedex 08, France

© International Agency for Research on Cancer 1988

All rights reserved. No part of this publication may be reproduced,
stored in a retrieval system or transmitted, in any form or by any means,
electronic, mechanical, photocopying, recording, or otherwise,
without the prior permission of the copyright holder.

ISBN 92 832 1415 3

CONTENTS

SECTION I

Description of On-Going or Planned Prospective Studies on Diet and Cancer

Saracci R.
  Prospective studies on diet and cancer:
  Reasons and opportunities for international collaboration 1

Willett W.C.
  Prospective studies of diet and cancer at Harvard University 12

van den Brandt P.A., Bausch-Goldbohm R.A., van 't Veer P.,
Hermus R., Sturmans F.
  The Dutch prospective cohort study on diet and cancer 18

Collette H.J.A., Baanders-van Halewejin A, de Waard F., Rombach J.J.,
van Noord P.A.H.
  Logistical aspects of longitudinal studies, with collection and
  storage of biological samples 28

Berrino F., Pisani P., Muti P., Crosignani P., Panico S., Pierotti M.,
Secreto G., Totis A., Fissi R., Mazzoleni C.
  Prospective study of hormones and diet in the etiology of
  breast cancer 34

Clavel F., Doyon F., Flamant R.
  Ideas for a possible prospective study on subjects belonging to
  a health insurance plan in Paris 39

Pietinen P., Virtamo J., Huttunen J.K.
  Overview of prospective studies on diet, cancer and
  cardiovascular diseases in Finland 41

Lindgärde F.
  Contribution of population screening programmes for the
  recruitment of subjects to be followed prospectively 45

Ewertz, M.
  Plans for a prospective study on diet and cancer in Denmark 50

Boeing H., Wahrendorf J., Thiel C., Heinemann L., Kulesza W.,
Rywik S.L., Sznajd J.
  Preliminary results from a feasibility study assessing the
  comparability of dietary information collected in different
  population surveys for possible use in a pooled cohort study on
  the occurrence of cancer 53

SECTION II

Dietary Assessment Methods for Epidemiological Studies

Pietinen P.
    Methodological study for the validation of two self-administered dietary questionnaires in Finland. Results and practical implications for epidemiological studies 63

Kaldor J.
    The problem of measurement error in cancer epidemiology with particular reference to cohort studies of diet 65

Willett W.C.
    Reproducibility and validity of a self-administered dietary questionnaire 71

Bausch-Goldbohm R.A., van den Brandt P.A., van 't Veer P., Sturmans F., Hermus R.J.J.
    Results of the methodological study for the design of a simplified, self-administered questionnaire 79

Crosignani P., Mazzoleni C.
    Comparison of dietary habits estimated either by food frequency or food frequency combined with portion size 90

SECTION III

Biochemical, Anthropometric and Other Objective Measures of Diet and Nutritional Status

Renaud S., Martin J.L.
    Biochemical indicators of fat intake and the risk of cardiovascular disease 101

van Noord P.A.H., Collette H.J.A., de Waard F. Rombach J.J.
    Caloric restriction in early life; effects on breast cancer risk factors? (The DOM based Dutch famine study) 112

Panico S.
    Anthropometric measurements in relation to hormonal patterns and breast cancer 120

SECTION IV

Prospective Studies on Cancer in Relation to Endogenous and Exogenous Hormones

Berrino F., Muti P., Pisani P.
    Overview of the etiological hypotheses linking endogenous
    steroid hormones and breast cancer 125

Key, T.J.A.
    Exogenous sex hormones and cancer: Recent findings on sex
    hormone binding globulin, risk factors for breast cancer, and
    oral contraceptives 143

Trichopoulos D., Petridou E.
    Exogenous determinants of pregnancy oestrogens and their
    relevance to cancer etiology. A study in Greece 146

Ewertz, M.
    Hormones and cancer multiple primary cancers of the female
    reproductive organs 157

SECTION I

Description of On-Going or Planned
Prospective Studies on Diet and Cancer

PROSPECTIVE STUDIES ON DIET AND CANCER: REASONS AND OPPORTUNITIES FOR INTERNATIONAL COLLABORATION

R. Saracci

International Agency for Research on Cancer, 150 cours Albert Thomas
69372 Lyon Cedex 08, France

Two of the principal investigators of the Framingham study wrote once: "No doubt there are nearly as many rationales for prospective studies as there are investigators using the method" (Gordon and Kannel, 1972). Maybe that is a less light statement than it appears to be at first, and has the advantage of putting to rest any further discussion. Still, one might venture some considerations on why prospective studies on the relationship between diet and cancer or, more correctly, cancers, are necessary at this juncture in time: this being the real issue, rather than the necessity in an abstract sense. One may gauge the timeliness of such studies by reference to the specific diet-cancer hypotheses nowadays under debate (a topic which will be addressed by several speakers at this meeting) or, more generally, in respect to the foreseeable yield of the prospective approach, as it can be assessed by briefly replying to three questions:

1. To what extent have cohort studies, prospective or historical, already contributed critical information to clarifying the aetiology of cancer?

2. To what extent have cohort studies already contributed critical information in other major areas of public health interest, for example, in cardiovascular diseases?

3. What are the main advantages that we can expect today from prospective studies on diet and cancer?

1. <u>To what extent have cohort studies, prospective or historical, already contributed critical information to the clarification of the aetiology of cancer?</u>

One way of answering is by looking at the summary of the IARC Monographs Programme on the Evaluation of the Carcinogenic Risk of Chemicals to Humans. Since 1972 this programme has been evaluating the carcinogenicity of single chemicals, groups of chemicals, industrial processes and occupational exposures (and is presently moving - January 1987 - to consider a broader spectrum of exposures, single or complex, outside the domain of chemicals). For each agent a separate evaluation is first made of the available experimental data, mainly carcinogenicity tests in animals, and of the human data, on the basis of which an overall evaluation and categorization is then made. Supplement 4 to the Monographs Series presents the results of the evaluation for all the agents previously considered in detail and published in Volumes 1 - 29 of the series. Agents assigned to Category 1 are those evaluated as definitely carcinogenic to humans, namely, those for which the evidence for carcinogenicity obtained directly from studies in humans is judged "sufficient" by itself (and, in principle, it could stand alone even if no other evidence from the laboratory were to be available). It can be seen from Table 1 that for a very high percentage of agents in this category cohort study data have contributed to the evidence in humans. The percentage remains substantial, but lower for Category 2 agents (agents probably carcinogenic to humans). The last column of the table shows a clear and marked gradient indicating an association between the level of confidence in evaluating and declaring an agent carcinogenic to man and the availability of data coming from cohort studies. This on one side substantiates the key role of cohort studies data in building up the assessment of the evidence, and on the other hand falls completely into line with the orthodox textbook doctrine according to which the strength of evidence of causality increases, going from correlation studies to case-control studies to cohort studies and, within these, from those purely observational to the experimental ones. If, instead of looking to all carcinogens as in Table 1, one restricts attention to the major carcinogens in terms of impact, the relevance of cohort studies is unchanged or perhaps even increases. For such major agents as tobacco, alcohol, hepatitis B virus, ionizing radiations and, within the occupational field, asbestos and aromatic amines, not only are there extensive cohort studies data available, but often data from prospective cohort studies or from historical studies which become prospective at a given point in time. These studies have often contributed, in a unique way, quantitative information on exposure-response relationships, including the temporal aspects.

From this bird's eye view it emerges that cohort studies have and are generating key information for the identification of agents causing cancers and for the quantification of their role. However, it is of interest to note that, as of today, none of the well-established carcinogenic agents is a dietary component, with the exception of aflatoxin (which is a food contaminant).

2. **To what extent have cohort studies already contributed critical information in other major areas of public health interest, for example, in cardiovascular diseases?**

Cardiovascular diseases, in particular ischaemic heart disease (IHD) represent the topic on which prospective epidemiological studies, now regarded as classic, have concentrated, starting soon after World War II. An attitude of caution and doubt on what it would be possible to achieve through other approaches, notably case-control studies, appears to have soon dominated the way of thinking in this area of research, leading to the inception of cohort studies on one side and to the quick shelving of the case-control approach on the other. However, some early case-control comparisons, though rather rudimentary in design, had pointed in a fruitful direction. For instance, already in 1950-51 Gertler et al., described elevated serum levels of total, free and esterified cholesterol (as well as of phospholipids and uric acid) in myocardial infarction patients in respect to healthy subjects (Gertler et al., 1951), while no correlation was found between dietary cholesterol and serum cholesterol in either patients or controls (Gertler et al., 1950).

The main reasons for regarding case-control studies as an inadequate tool and, at the best, only as a screening device for picking up risk factors, have been summarized by A. Keys (1966): "Comparison of coronary heart disease patients with apparently healthy counterparts is a classical clinico-epidemiological approach, well exemplified by the study by Gertler, White et al., on young 'coronaries' (1954). Such comparisons yield clues and theories but nothing certain about risk prediction. Since the first attack kills one-third of the patients within a few days, comparisons are limited to the less interesting group, the survivors. Moreover, for some of the variables of interest, the characteristics of the patients are certainly the result of the clinical disease and so could not be useful in predicting the predisease risk. Finally, any control group is bound to include many persons who have advanced but silent coronary heart disease". While these methodological remarks have a maximum bearing for variables like blood pressure, concentrations of hormones or of physiological chemicals with a potential pathogenic role, they also apply to a variable like diet, as it is measurable in case-control investigations. This is an aspect pertinent to diet-cancer studies as well, as are, on the other hand, some of the features which have characterized the development of prospective studies on IHD. I will enlist here four pertinent features.

First, as already mentioned, prospective studies were started very early - as soon as a few initial clues to putative aetiological factors of IHD were available, less copious and documented than the dietary clues now in hand for cancer at some sites like colon, rectum and breast. This early start was not without weaknesses in study design and implementation. The Framingham study was launched in 1948 by the U.S. Public Health Service and enrollment went on between 1949 and 1952. The initial response of the selected sample of subjects aged 30-59 was, in the words of the investigators (Gordon and Kannel, 1972), "poor" (68.8%) and "biased": the responders appeared healthier than the non-responders and this bias was reinforced by the addition of a sizable group of even healthier volunteers. As the exposure-disease relationship may differ between responders and non-responders the best way of ensuring that a distortion has not occurred is by having the relationship observed among responders confirmed by other similar studies (which proved true for several of the key results of the Framingham study). Susser (1985), commenting on the post-World War II development of the prospective study approach in the U.S., remarks that: "Yet today, if one is to judge by the initial protocols referred to in various accounts of its history, the Framingham Study could not hope to be funded". Have scientific standards in epidemiology become higher or just more "standard", that is, stiflingly conformistic?

The second noteworthy feature in the development of the prospective investigations of IHD was that confirmation of findings was made possible by the availability of multiple studies, some starting about the same time as the Framingham project or soon afterwards, others being added during nearly two decades. Table 2 (adapted from Keys (1980)), shows a selection of major studies (for some of them the total number of subjects enrolled exceeded the number in the specific subset of interest indicated in the table). The size of the groups studied ranges from a few hundred subjects to several thousands as the maximum. It took 10 to 15 years from the start of the first investigation to the full "recognition of the requirement of large numbers, beyond those available in any one study, to evaluate with a reasonable level of certainty the relationship of several traits to risk of coronary heart disease". This prompted the formation of a "Pooling Project Research Group" which ultimately was able to combine data from five major prospective studies within the United States (Pooling Project Research Group, 1978). The requirement of large study populations is going to be much more serious for cancer studies, as even the most common cancers entail a frequency of observable "events" (cancer cases or deaths) substantially lower than IHD, particularly if the assessment of the latter includes not only deaths but also softer end-points clinically or electrocardiographically measurable. As a rough estimate changing the primary focus of investigation from IHD to a common cancer (lung, stomach, colon-rectum) involves changing the size of the population to be followed up by an order of magnitude, from several thousand to several tens of thousands up to the hundred thousands.

A third feature of prospective studies on IHD is the development of studies across nations. Not only were studies carried out in different countries, but the element of international comparison has been the central feature of one of the best known studies, the "Seven Countries". The dimensions of the study are indicated in Table 3, which reports for each of the populations involved in the "Seven Countries" the number of coronary events (deaths and definite myocardial infarctions) as assessed at the 10 year follow-up. Figures 1 and 2, in which each circle represents one population, exemplifies some of the relationships found in the study: that of cholesterol _versus_ dietary intake of fats (saturated and polyunsaturated) and that of dietary intake of saturated fat _versus_ coronary events incidence. Unlike the relationship between cholesterol and HID incidence (already emerging from the initial follow-up in Framingham, Table 4 (Dawber et al., 1957), and confirmed again and again by later evidence) these two relationships have been most difficult to demonstrate convincingly at the individual level, as opposed to the population level to which Figures 1 and 2 refer. The difficulty appears to stem from: (a) the amount of intraindividual variation in dietary intake which is capable, lest special care and repeated measurements are used, of obscuring the inter-individual variation in diet intake; and (b) presumably, the coexistence of important (genetic?) differences between individuals in handling dietary components, so that to the same level of dietary intake of saturated fat and cholesterol corresponds a sizable spectrum of blood cholesterol levels. Ultimately, both factors would contribute to dilute until the point of undetectability any relationship between dietary components and IHD incidence rates (unless, as some authors (Oliver, 1987) are still inclined to believe, the general relevance of the relationship between diet and IHD should be genuinely doubted).

Certainly, and this is the fourth noteworthy feature of the IHD prospective studies, without the comparative data from different populations the balance of the evidence would today be much less favourable to the diet-IHD hypothesis, and this notwithstanding the mass of observations accruing from the prospective studies and, more recently, from intervention trials. As it may well be that the diet-cancer associations to be discovered entail increases in risk of the same magnitude as for the cholesterol-IHD association (say twofold-threefold between upper and lower fifths of the distribution of cholesterol within a certain population), this lesson from the IHD studies is strictly relevant to the planning of diet-cancer investigations: and this in terms of methods to assess habitual dietary intake and biological markers, size of the populations to be studied, and variability in intake within and, most important, _between_ the populations selected for long-term study.

3. **What are the main advantages that we can expect today from prospective studies on diet and cancer?**

I will briefly look only on the bright side here, namely the potential advantages of prospective studies, this being the necessary prerequirement of any further discussion weighing advantages against costs. Prospective studies on diet and cancer, particularly those of longitudinal type, namely involving repeated examinations of the study subjects, offer opportunities:

1. to investigate the natural history of the disease, from early indicators of exposure to preclinical lesions to clinical cancer;

2. to reduce selection bias, a feature shared by other population-based studies, for instance, population-based case-control studies;

3. to reduce observation bias, as exposure measurements (on diet) are taken before the occurrence of cancer;

4. to perform repeat measurements of exposures with the aim of improving accuracy of measurements (thus reducing misclassification of subjects) and of identifying time changes potentially relevant to disease development;

5. to interpret more confidently "small" (say in the range 1.5 - 3) relative risks;

6. to improve the study of interactions.

These potential advantages of prospective studies, not shared by other types of epidemiological investigations, stand on the premise that an "explanatory" approach to diet and cancer is both warranted and needed, focused on identifying and quantifying the pathogenic or protective role of specific nutrients, food items and food groups. The alternative and, if brought to the extreme, opposite approach has the purely "pragmatic" aim of identifying feasible diet changes and to quantitate associated variations in cancer risks. Though an attractive short-cut to prevention, the latter may easily end, as short cuts often do, in a blind alley, as the specific dietary components responsible for the observed changes in cancer risk cannot be defined with confidence. At its best the pragmatic approach generates results of local value for the population where they were obtained, which are, however, very problematic to extrapolate to other populations. The experience in the IHD area indicates that essentially pragmatic preventive trials ("second generation" trials) attempting to modify several major risk factors simultaneously could not have been conceived, nor their results subsequently interpreted, without the wealth of information previously derived from the long-term prospective studies. Faced with the present hypotheses for the dietary aetiology of several major cancers and with the corresponding lack of any firm evidence of real causation, going into pragmatic studies and side-stepping prospective observational studies appears like a leap into the dark. This may have serious consequences on our ability to understand the role of dietary factors in cancer and our ability to soundly base our preventive actions. The issue is not understanding as an exercise in academic purism, but for the needs of effective prevention. Whether "pragmatic" intervention studies on diet and cancer are justified today may be a moot point, but that prospective "explanatory" studies are required is scarcely debatable. Collaboration between studies may enhance their information yield and may even be essential to obviate limitations, for instance in population size, intrinsic to each individual study. In the first place, one may hope that this collaboration, whatever its form, starts earlier than turned out to be possible withthe IHD studies. Indeed, one may wish that it go hand in hand with the development of the individual studies, if at all possible from their planning phase. As sketched in Table 5, between a true multicentric study, in which most methodological elements are planned and kept in common throughout all the population groups (often located far apart) included in the study, and a combined study, typified by an <u>a posteriori</u> formal or informal meta-analysis, stands a "coordinated" study in which some common elements are identified early in the development of the studies. It is at this level that collaboration between the different research groups conducting prospective studies on diet and cancer can be set up. The variety of objectives, method and local circumstances makes wholly unrealistic the idea of a multicentric study. On the other hand, it would be wasteful of resources if in 10 or 20 years time, when results flow in, the possibility of combining findings on a number of diet-cancer questions would be frustrated by differences between studies which could have been prevented inexpensively if recognized and dealt with by collaborative action at earlier stages. A major objective of this meeting is to start to identify differences and common elements between ongoing and planned studies in several areas, which I enlist here - for the sake of our discussions - as suggestions for collaboration:

1. Methodology for dietary assessment.

2. Methodology and objectives for the creation and/or use of biological banks.

3. Combination of questionnaire-based studies with data from existing biological banks.

4. Inter-centre cooperation on methodology and techniques for hormone determinations.

5. Collaborative studies on rare cancers for which no single study can provide a sufficient number of cases.

6. Collaborative studies on rare exposures such as consumption of particular food items, specific dietary habits (e.g. vegetarians), use of particular drugs (e.g., oral contraceptives), etc.

7. Collaborative studies on common hypotheses which can be tested by means of a multicentric approach.

8. Use of prospective studies on cancer for the investigation of other disease end-points (e.g., cardiovascular, metabolic).

The International Agency for Research on Cancer offers today the small contribution of this, hopefully, timely meeting to explore the potential for collaboration. Should we all agree that this potential is worth exploiting, the Agency is ready to operate as an instrument towards this collective end.

REFERENCES

Dawber, T.R., Moore, F.E., Mann, G.V. (1957) Coronary heart disease in the Framingham Study. Am. J. Publ. Hlth, 47, 4-24

Gertler, M.M., Garn, S.M., & White, P.D. (1950) Diet, serum cholesterol and coronary heart disease. Circulation, 2, 696

Gertler, M.M. & White, P.D. (1954) Coronary heart disease in young adults. A multidisciplinary study. Harvard University Press, Cambridge, Massachusetts

Gertler, M.M., Driskell, M.M., Bland, E.F., Garn, S.M., Lerman, J., Levine, S.A., Sprague, H.B. & White, P.D. (1951) Clinical aspects of coronary heart disease: an analysis of 100 cases in patients 23 to 40 years of age with myocardial infarction. J.A.M.A., 146, 1291-1295

Gordon, T. & Kannel, W.B. (1972) The prospective study of cardiovascular disease. In: Stewart, G.T., ed, Trends in Epidemiology, Charles C. Thomas, Springfield, Illinois, pp. 189-211

Keys, A. (1966) The individual risk of coronary heart disease. Ann. N.Y. Acad. Sci., 134, 1046-1056

Keys, A. (1980) Seven Countries, a multivariate analysis of death and coronary heart disease, Harvard University Press, Cambridge, Massachusetts

Oliver, M. (1987) Diet and coronary heart disease. Health Trends, 19, 8-11

Pooling Project Research Group (1978) Relationship of blood pressure, serum cholesterol, smoking habit, relative weight and ECG abnormalities to incidence of major coronary events: final report of the pooling project. J. Chron. Dis., 31, 201-306

Susser, M. (1985) Epidemiology in the United States after World War II: the evolution of technique. Epidemiol. Reviews, 7, 147-177

Table 1. Cohort study data available for agents classified as definitely or probably carcinogenic to humans*

Agent class	No. of agents	No. of agents with cohort study data	Percent of agents with cohort study data
Definitely carcinogenic to humans:			
- industrial processes and occupational exposures	7	7	100
- chemicals and groups of chemicals	23	21	91
Probably carcinogenic to humans:			
- higher probability	14	10	71
- lower probability	47	26	55

* IARC Monographs Volumes 1 - 29.

Table 2. Major prospective studies on men aged 40-59

Study	Year of entry	Number	Response rate (%)
1. Minnesota business, professional men 45-55	1948	300	92
2. Framingham residents 40-60+	1948-50	1,379	66
3. Los Angeles civil servants	1950-51	1,092	75
4. San Francisco longshoremen, 35-64	1951	3,263	67
5. Albany, N.Y. civil servants	1953-54	1,829	89
6. Chicago Western Electric Co. employees	1957	2,080	67
7. Chicago Peoples Gas Co. employees	1958	1,465	92
8. Tecumseh, Michigan, residents	1959-60	798	88
9. California corporation employees, 39-59	1960	3,524	66
10. Oslo, Norway, employees, 40-49	1960	3,751	?
11. Evans County, Georgia, residents, 45-64	1960-62	646	92
12. Gothenburg, Sweden, men born 1913, aged 50	1963	855	88
13. Israel civil servants	1963	7,666	86
14. Two areas of Yugoslavia, residents, 35-62	1964-68	11,121	93
15. Puerto Rico residents, 45-59	1965-68	6,954	81
16. Japanese in Honolulu, residents, 45-59	1965-68	6,217	81

Table 3. The "Seven Countries" study – 10 year incidence
(Hard CHD = CHD deaths or definite myocardial infarction)

Cohort	Number	All-causes	CHD deaths	Hard CHD
U.S. railroad*	2,571	294	146	–
Dalmatia	671	61	7	14
Slavonia	696	124	15	22
Tanushimaru	508	58	5	9
East Finland	817	147	78	115
West Finland	860	127	30	61
Ushibuka	502	70	4	13
Crevalcore	993	136	24	51
Montegiorgio	719	74	10	27
Zutphen	878	109	38	59
Crete	686	42	1	4
Corfu	529	43	8	19
Rome railroad**	768	77	22	31
Velika Krsna	511	63	4	8
Zrenjanin	516	60	8	14
Belgrade	538	27	13	19
Total	12,763	1,512	413	466

* No 10-year examinations
** Ten-year examinations incomplete

Table 4. ASHD in the first four years of follow-up, Framingham males, age 45-62 (1957)

Cholesterol (per 100 ml)	Population	New cases	Rate/1000	Relative rate
≥ 260 mg	131	16	122	2.90
225 - 259	188	8	42	1.08
< 225	334	13	39	1.00

Table 5.

Collaborative (composite) study	Elements in common between individual (component) studies			
	Hypotheses	Design & methods	Analyses	A priori planning
Multicentric	Most	Most	Most	Yes
Coordinated	Some	Some	Some	Yes
Combined	Some	Some	Some	No

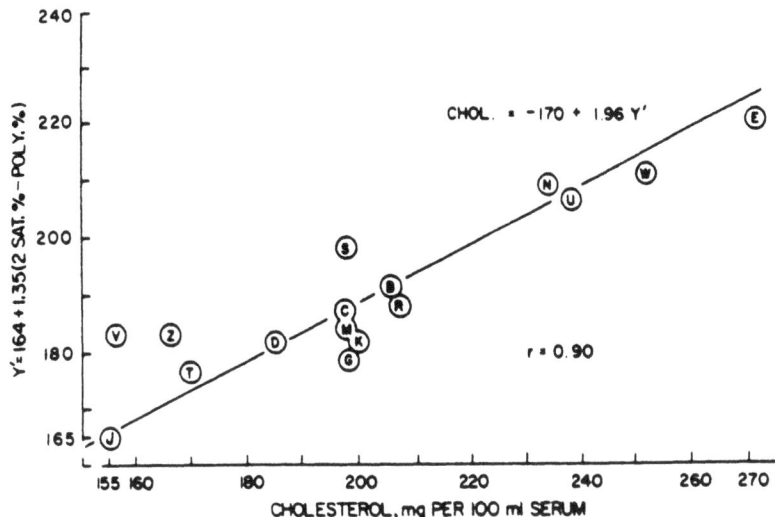

Figure 1. Relation of mean serum cholesterol concentration of the cohorts at entry to fat composition of the diet expressed in the multiple regression equation derived from controlled dietary experiments in Minnesota. B = Belgrade; C = Crevalcore; D = Dalmatia; E = east Finland; G = Corfu; J = Ushibuka; K = Crete; M = Montegiorgio; N = Zutphen; R = Rome railroad; S = Slavonia; T = Tanushimaru; U = American railroad; V = Velika Krsna; W = west Finland; Z = Zrenjanin.

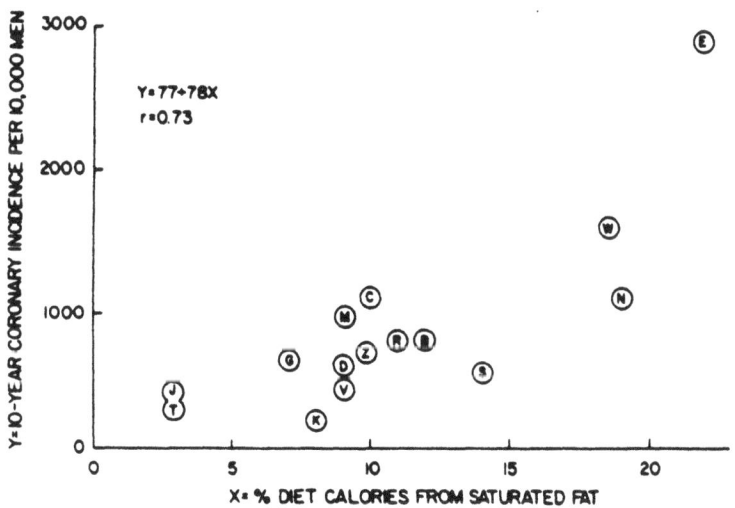

Figure 2. Ten-year incidence rate of coronary heart disease, by any diagnostic criterion, plotted against the percentage of dietary calories supplied by saturated fatty acids. Cohorts as in figure 1.

PROSPECTIVE STUDIES OF DIET AND CANCER AT HARVARD UNIVERSITY

W.C. Willett

Harvard School of Public Health, Channing Laboratory, 180 Longwood Avenue, Boston, MA 02115, USA

INTRODUCTION

While we are engaged in the conduct of several case-control studies of diet and cancer, our research group is concentrating its efforts on prospective studies of their relationship. Case-control studies certainly will continue to play a role in elucidating the relation between dietary factors and cancer incidence. However, the potential for bias related to the selection of controls (since participation rates are declining and are often between 60 and 70%) and the recall of past diet by patients ill with cancer may render the interpretation of findings from these investigations less reliable. We therefore tend to feel more confident about findings based on the prospective studies than we do about data derived from our case-control studies.

I will discuss three specific prospective studies:
1) The Nurses Health Study, which has been ongoing since 1976,
2) The Health Professionals Follow-up Study, a recently started study among men using many of the same methods that have been learned in the conduct of the Nurses Health Study, and
3) The Physicians Health Study, which is a randomized, double-blind trial.
This presentation will focus on the Nurses Health Study because it has provided our longest experience.

The Nurses Health Study

This study, whose principal investigator is Frank Speizer, began in 1976. At that time, we mailed questionnaires to all married female registered nurses who were between 30 and 35 years of age and residing in 11 large states within the United States. About 70% of those receiving a questionnaire mailed them back, yielding a total of 121 700 women. This study was initially established primarily to examine oral contraceptives and post-menopausal estrogens in relation to reproductive cancers, primarily breast cancer. Also, a component was incorporated within this same cohort to examine cardiovascular outcomes.

Follow-up of the cohort is conducted every two years by mailing a questionnaire to all participants. These questionnaires are used both to update exposure information (for example, we ask about current use of oral contraceptives, post-menopausal estrogens, weight, smoking status, and a wide variety of other exposures) and to ascertain outcome events. The questionnaire includes a list of diseases, and participants are asked to report whether or not they have had these diagnosed in the two-year interval since the last questionnaire and, if so, to provide and data and (for some diagnoses) further details.

The nutritional component of the Nurses Health Study began in 1980 when the scope of our questionnaire was expanded considerably to include a dietary questionnaire that was mailed to the cohort. We have called this a semiquantitative food frequency questionnaire. It included a list of 61 food items that were carefully selected, using step-wise regression analysis of a longer questionnaire, to be the most discriminating for 18 nutrients of specific interest. About 98 000 women returned the dietary questionnaire in 1980.

After the 1982 questionnaire, we asked women to send a sample of their toenail clippings. These were primarily collected for selenium analysis; however, we are now using them for the analysis of a wide variety of elements. At least for selenium, nails seem to be a very useful measure that provides an unusual time integration for selenium intake. These nails have been catalogued, and we are using them for nested case-control studies of selenium in relation to cancer.

In 1984 we modified our dietary questionnaire, which is now expanded in length to include about 120 food items. The capacity to increase the size of the dietary questionnaire was partly based on the use of optical scanning technology, since we had been limited in the number of questions we could ask by the data entry costs. In 1982 we converted to optical scanning for data entry; this allowed us to collect more data at much reduced cost. The expanded dietary questionnaire was mailed in the 1984 and 1986 follow-up cycles. Questionnaires are printed on continuous, optically scannable paper. We print names and addresses on the forms and also imprint identification numbers in both a directly readable format and a machine readable format. This provides a fail-safe link between name and ID number. We are now planning to convert to a four-year cycle of diet assessment rather than a two-year cycle; thus we will be mailing our food frequency questionnaires again in 1990.

Although the Nurses Health Study was primarily designed as a cancer study, we are also examining all major cardiovascular end-points, including myocardial infarction, stroke, pulmonary embolism, and sudden death. We recently began a detailed study of the etiology of type 2 non-insulin dependent diabetes. We now have over 1 000 incident cases in the cohort. We are also looking at rheumatoid arthritis, lupus, erythematosus, gall bladder disease, and a variety of other outcomes.

End-points are initially self-reported, but we carefully document each report using various methods. For some diagnoses we have shown that a supplementary questionnaire requesting further details of the diagnosis is sufficient. This may be true because all women in the study are nurses, who were chosen as a study population because it was thought that their self-reports would be unusually accurate. For diabetes, as an example, we have an additional one-page questionnaire on which we request details about blood sugar levels over time. This questionnaire has been validated in a subsample in which we actually obtained the blood sugar reports; these substantiated the self-reports of blood sugar levels to a high degree. Therefore, for the total group of diabetics this supplementary questionnaire is sufficient (and far less costly than obtaining medical records). For all cancers (except non-melanoma skin cancer) we request pathology reports, and for melanoma we actually obtain tissue blocks since we found that about a third of the pathology reports that specify melanoma are not substantiated when the blocks are reviewed by one pathologist.

For each two-year follow-up cycle we generally receive quetsionnaires back from about 85-90% of the cohort after up to five mailing to non-respondents. In 1982 we telephoned the non-respondents; this provided a 94% follow-up with actual contact at the six-year point.

Mortality in the cohort is ascertained by use of the National Death Index (Stampfer et al., 1984), which is a computerized listing of deaths within the United States. We also learn about roughly two-thirds of deaths by report from families or the postal system when we mail out a follow-up questionnaire. With the mortality search we estimate that we have ascertained at least 96% of the deaths within the cohort.

The above describes very briefly the operation of the Nurses Health Study. This generates a very large amount of data, so that the data management has been a continuing and growing challenge for us. The optical scanning technology, which began in 1982 as noted above, has been very useful. We conducted several pilot studies to be certain that it was sufficiently accurate; it proved more accurate than manual key entry of data. The optically scanned format has also proved to be more acceptable to the subjects in the study than our previous, more unstructured questionnaires. Computing costs for the study were high; we were running well over US $100 000 a year for computing and were still not able to conduct all the required analyses. More recently, we bought our own computers and now we have several dedicated to this project. We never have quite enough storage space for data; however, this is a chronic problem for a study that continually adds large amounts of information each year.

As an example of data based on the Nurses Health Study, I will describe an analysis related to the primary dietary hypothesis at the beginning of the study, that fat intake is positively associated with risk of breast cancer (Willett et al., 1987a). This hypothesis is based largely on animal studies and international correlations; there have been only a few case-control studies of this relationship.

Our validation study will be discussed in more detail later in this meeting; however, it needs to be mentioned now since it provides a key to the interpretation of the data based on a total cohort. One basic question is: what is the actual distribution of fat intake in this population? Based on 28 days of diet record per subject among women in the validation study, we found that the mean of the lowest quintile was 32% of calories from fat whereas the mean of the highest quintile was 44% of calories from fat. Now that, of course, is not as large a range of fat intake as one would like to study, but it does correspond roughly to current recommendations to reduce fat intake from about 40% of calories (the average USA intake) to about 30%. Thus our study is a fair test of the current dietary recommendations. For specific types of fats the variation is somewhat greater; for saturated fat the lowest quintile was about 11% of calories and the highest quintile was about 17% of calories. After excluding questionnaires with ten or more blanks on the food items (4%), those with extreme values (2.5%), and women with a previous diagnosis of cancer (2.5%), 85 538 women with complete dietary information and no previous history of cancer remained.

For these analyses, we used breast cancer cases that were diagnosed after the return of the 1980 questionnaire but before 1 June 1984, which was our four-year follow-up questionnaire. We obtained pathology records for 91% of these self-reported cases; 99% of these self-reported cases were confirmed by the pathology reports that we obtained. We divided women into quintiles according to their fat inake and calculated age-adjusted relative risks, with the lowest fat intake quintile as the referent. The hypothesis was not confirmed; in fact, there was a trend that was almost statistically significant in the opposite direction. We adjusted one at a time and simultaneously for known risk factors for breast cancer; this made very little difference. the 95% confidence interval (0.64-1.05) around the point estimate (0.82) for the highest level of calorie-adjusted total fat intake included one, but in fact the upper bound of the confidence interval, with this large sample size, was only slightly above unity, providing fairly strong evidence that there is not an important positive association between dietary fat intake within this range.

In addition to total fat intake, we examined saturated fat, linoleic acid and cholesterol intake; similar weak inverse relationships were seen for each of these components. We also explored many subgroups; in none was there any hint of a positive association. Pre-menopausal <u>versus</u> post-menopausal breast cancer was of particular interest; the findings were similarly inverse for both.

In contrast to dietary fat, the association of alcohol intake with risk of breast cancer was quite clear in this study (Willett <u>et al.</u>, 1987b). At a low alcohol intake there was really no increase in risk compared with non-drinkers; this is quite important because it means that there is not something strange about teetotallers that makes them at low risk of breast cancer. However, for 5 g to 14.9 g a day the relative risk was 1.3. This is only about 3-9 drinks of alcohol per week. For 15 g a day or more, which is a little over a drink a day, the relative risk was 1.6. The test for trend was highly significant. This association with alcohol is not a unique finding; there are four prospective studies in which this relationship has been examined and it has been seen in all four. There are also now about nine case-control studies, including several from France and Italy, in which a positive association has been seen. This is turning out to be a remarkably consistent finding; in fact it is the only reasonably consistent dietary association with breast cancer risk at this time.

The Health Professionals Follow-up Study

This is our effort to conduct a study among a population of men similar to the one we are doing among women in the Nurses Health Study. We have continued the use of health professional groups for study populations, which has proved to be very successful in the context of the Nurses Health Study. We have therefore enrolled dentists, veterinarians, podiatrists, optometrists and several other smaller groups of health professionals to obtain enough men, since no single group had a large enough membership. The study is funded by the National Heart, Lung and Blood Institute. In the first five years, our statistical power for most cancers is going to be a little bit weak; however, there will be well over one thousand myocardial infarctions. This may be a useful strategy; to use a prospective study during the first five years primarily for heart disease outcomes, and beyond that time for both heart disease and cancer. Study participants are between the ages of 40 and 75 years, which is a bit older than the nurses, so that many end-points will accumulate just as rapidly as in our study among women. Our exposure data, as for the nurses, is based on mailed questionnaires which are very similar to those used in the Nurses Health Study. We are also collecting nails from the men for elemental analyses. At this point in time we have enrolled about 44 000 men; ultimately we hope to have around 50 000 participants in this cohort.

The Physicians Health Study

This study, which is conducted under the direction of Charlie Hennekens, is a randomized, double-blind trial to evaluate the hypothesis that beta-carotene, consumed at the dose of 30 mg on alternate days, can reduce the incidence of cancer at all sites combined (Stampfer <u>et al.</u>, 1985). A second hypothesis being evaluated is that aspirin consumed as a single tablet (approximately 300 mg) on alternate days can reduce death due to cardiovascular disease. Both hypotheses are being evaluated simultaneously using a two-by-two factorial design. This study will be discussed only briefly since it is probably not quite so relevant to the topic of the meeting.

Study subjects are U.S. male physicians, 40 or more years of age. At this point in time, randomization is complete and nearly 22 000 physicians have been enrolled. Follow-up is now approaching five years for those that were enrolled at the very beginning. Both morbidity and mortality follow-up is quite complete; this is a very stable group of people that are relatively easy to track. Compliance remains extremely high in this study, partly due to the fact that there was a six-month run-in period during which subjects were all given the same pills or capsules to evaluate adherence to protocol. Almost one third of run-in participants dropped out during this time before randomization, so that compliance after randomization has been excellent.

At baseline, blood samples were collected by mail from about 16 000 participants. These were aliquoted and frozen at $-80°C$. Nested case-control studies are now being conducted using these blood samples to address a variety of hypotheses related both to heart disease and cancer.

CONCLUSIONS

I believe that these prospective studies, together, will allow us to address a very wide variety of hypotheses over the coming years. We have already had an opportunity to examine a number of factors in relation to breast cancer, and are still exploring some additional factors possibly associated with this disease. Prospective studies do help us keep our priorities straight. We necessarily examine the common malignancies first, and the uncommon cancers are appropriately analyzed last, since they accumulate over a longer period of time. Although we will learn much in these studies, it is important to point out that they have limitations. For example, we cannot look at levels of dietary intake outside the ranges of exposure within the United States. It certainly would be interesting to know the effect of 20% of calories from fat intake on risk of breast cancer. However, this is something that we simply cannot determine within the context of these particular studies, since very few people in the United States consume such a diet. Similarly, we will not be able to study uncommon tumours, at least in the short run; this is one reason to consider pooling data from multiple prospective studies. Furthermore, we are not sure that it will be possible to study the effects of diet early in life. We have asked about diet during the high school years on our last questionnaire, but it is not clear how valid these data are; others are conducting studies on this issue.

It seems likely that the studies I have described will yield many interesting findings over the next few years. Yet, they will not provide data over the entire range of possible human intake or provide data about the possible effects of diet at all periods in life. It will, therefore, be important to conduct studies in various environments and over long periods of time to expand our understanding of the relation of diet with human cancer.

REFERENCES

Stampfer, M.J., Willett, W.C., Speizer, F.E., et al. (1984) Test of the National Death Index. Am. J. Epidemiol., 119, 836-839

Stampfer, M.J., Buring, J.E., Willett, W.C., Rosner, B., Eberlein, K. & Hennekens, C.H. (1985) The 2x2 factorial design: its application to a randomized trial of aspirin and carotene in U.S. physicians. Statistics in Medicine, 4, 111-116

Willett, W.C., Stampfer, M.J., Colditz, G.A., Rosner, B., Hennekens, C.H. & Speizer, F.E. (1987a) Dietary fat and the risk of breast cancer. N. Engl. J. Med., 316, 22-28

Willett, W.C., Stampfer, M.J., Colditz, G.A., Rosner, B., Hennekens, C.H. & Speizer, F.E. (1987b) Moderate alcohol consumption and risk of breast cancer. N. Engl. J. Med., 316, 1174-1180

THE DUTCH PROSPECTIVE COHORT STUDY ON DIET AND CANCER

P.A. van den Brandt[1], R.A. Bausch-Goldbohm[1,2], P. van 't Veer[2], R. Hermus[2] & F. Sturmans[1]

[1] Department of Epidemiology, University of Limburg, P.O. Box 616, 6200 MD Maastricht, The Netherlands

[2] TNO-CIVO Toxicology and Nutrition Institute, Zeist, The Netherlands

INTRODUCTION

A prospective cohort study on diet and cancer is currently being conducted in the Netherlands by the Department of Epidemiology of the University of Limburg at Maastricht and the Department of Human Nutrition of the TNO-CIVO Toxicology and Nutrition Institute at Zeist. External funding for the project is being provided by the Netherlands Cancer Foundation and the Ministry of Health.

The initial grant application in 1983 made it possible to carry out a two-year pilot study in 1984 and 1985. On the basis of the results of the pilot, the actual cohort study was started in 1986. The pilot project was proposed by our group to investigate the feasibility of the project and to develop the methods to be used in the cohort study. The results of this pilot study are expressed in the description of the cohort study that will follow. The description will be rather technical at various points, but this information might be of interest for other investigators who are planning similar prospective studies.

DESIGN

In view of the possible problems that are encountered when studying diet and cancer, such as intra- and inter-individual variability in food habits as well as various sorts of bias (selection bias, information bias), we proposed a prospective cohort study with the following features:
- The study will be conducted in a population whose dietary habits are relatively stable.
- Use will be made of an adequate dietary assessment method (questionnaire).
- The heterogeneity in the determinants will be enlarged by intentional overrepresentation of vegetarians.
- The questionnaire will be applied repeatedly to determine the stability of the food habits.

With the incorporation of these features, the cohort study was designed as follows. A sex-stratified random sample of the (general) Dutch population in the age range of 55-69 years will be obtained from municipal population registries. The aim was an initial sample size of 350,000, with equal numbers of men and women, to obtain a cohort of about 150,000 subjects. The choice of this age range was based on considerations of validity and efficiency. Younger age groups can be of interest for particular tumours, such as premenopausal breast cancer, but the assessment of dietary habits by questionnaire can be more difficult because the pattern may not yet have stabilized.

In older age groups dietary assessment also becomes more problematic (difficulties in completion), and there is a tendency to underreport and to have less histological verification for elderly cancer patients. Finally, with regard to financial constraints, research projects have to yield results within a usual funding period.

The baseline measurement of exposure will involve completion of a self-administered questionnaire on diet and other lifestyle factors, and the collection of toenail clippings.

In the years after baseline data collection, cancer follow-up of the cohort of respondents will be conducted by two types of tumour registries:
1) The National Cancer Registry, with its 8 participating Regional Cancer Registries.
2) PALGA, the National Data Base of Pathological Records, which is a pathology registry.

The cancer sites that will be studied initially are lung, stomach, colon, rectum and breast. These sites were chosen because they represent 67% of cancer mortality in the Netherlands (Central Bureau of Statistics, 1985), and nutrition is believed to play an important role in their causation.

Determinants

In the cohort study we will test the various prevailing hypotheses on the relation between diet and cancer that have been published in the literature. The questionnaire is therefore predominantly directed towards habitual intake of fat (various types), fibre, vitamins and their precursors, alcohol, cholesterol, nitrate and nitrite, sodium, selenium and synthetic antioxidants.

Apart from nutrients we will also look at risks associated with specific dietary patterns, since that opens possibilities in the area of prevention. A large part of the pilot study was devoted to the development of the questionnaire, and it is discussed in more detail by our colleague, R.A. Bausch-Goldbohm, elsewhere in this Report. A significant part of the questionnaire deals with the measurement of potential confounders of the diet-cancer relationship and other independent risk factors. These include: smoking history, occupation and socioeconomic status, history of selected medical conditions, family history of cancer, history of chronic drug use, history of oral contraceptive use and reproductive history, physical activity. As mentioned earlier, toenail clippings will be collected as well; these might give an indication of the long-term nutritional status of selenium and possibly other trace elements that might be of interest in cancer etiology.

We will now discuss in more detail the actual assembly of the cohort and the baseline exposure measurement.

Recruitment

With regard to recruitment of the study population we decided to make use of municipal population registries for reasons of efficiency and accuracy. Every citizen in the Netherlands is registered in a municipal registry in a very accurate way, and permission can be obtained to draw samples from these registries for research purposes. In view of the desired size of the study and cancer follow-up mechanisms, the municipalities participating were required to have a computerized population registry that could produce the selected samples on magnetic tape. Secondly, the degree of follow-up coverage needed to be sufficient in eligible municipalities.

With regard to the first requirement, we identified all the municipalities whose population registry was computerized through one of the 9 regional computing centres that provide services to municipalities. In addition, municipalities were identified that used their own computer system and were able to provide a population sample on tape. An initial survey was carried out among these 323 computerized municipalities (out of a total of 741), and 93% agreed to provide the requested population samples. Neither the computerization nor the participation is confined only to large municipalities.

Meanwhile, follow-up coverage according to municipality was also determined. In this case, we identified the pathology laboratories and hospitals that cooperate with the Cancer Registries and/or PALGA. The National Health Care Information Centre (SIG) provided data on the municipal origin of first admissions per diagnosis in these hospitals. On the basis of this information we were able to calculate, per cancer site, the expected coverage degree realized by these follow-up institutions.

By intersecting the list of municipalities and their corresponding coverage degrees with the list of computerized municipalities, we were able to construct various "cohorts" of different sizes depending on the desired minimal coverage degree of any municipality. The final choice involved a coverage cut-off point of 75%, yielding a tentative initial municipal sample of almost 350,000 people. The mean histological coverage degree would in this case be 93%. The location of the 205 municipalities that were chosen in this way is presented in Figure 1.

In an attempt to create more heterogeneity in the dietary habits of the cohort, we have actively recruited individuals with special dietary habits (vegetarians) in addition to the municipal sample. We defined "vegetarians" in this case as subjects eating meat less than twice a week. This recruitment involved advertisements and application forms in 5 selected magazines and 550 shops. Furthermore, a large producer of health food products agreed to enclose a number of application forms with two soya products. This active recruitment was concentrated on those areas of the country that are sufficiently covered with regard to cancer follow-up.

On the basis of earlier Dutch surveys we estimated that about 3% of the municipal sample would be in these special groups (according to our definition). We hoped to double this proportion in the cohort by intentional overrepresentation. During the period of recruitment (April-July 1986), approximately 1000 vegetarians applied for participation. Various applicants were considered ineligible because of age, place of residence (not living in areas covered by the survey) and other reasons, and finally 706 applications were retained.

After deciding that the survey for baseline data collection would be held in September 1986, we asked the cooperating municipalities to provide their lists by 1 May 1986. We realized that at the time of the survey a number of sampled subjects would have died or moved, but we anticipated that this long interval between selection and survey would be necessary. Problems indeed occurred with regard to timing of the samples, availability of selection packages and computer compatibility. These problems resulted in a modification of the sample size that was actually taken.

The municipal data were processed at the University of Limburg together with the vegetarian data, after which each subject was given an identification number. This ID number is printed on the questionnaire and will serve as the link between exposure data, disease data and personal identification data.

The size and origin of the recruited population is shown in Table 1. Due to the above-mentioned factors operating at the selection stage, the municipal sample was eventually drawn from 204 municipalities, and a total of 340,439 subjects were available. On every subject the following information was available: name, address, municipality of residence, data of birth and sex (social security number are not currently used in the Netherlands).

Distribution and collection

A tape containing the identification information was used to address and personalize the questionnaires that were subsequently distributed by mail in September 1986. Although we had originally planned to let the volunteers from the Netherlands Cancer Foundation participate by distributing and collecting the material (hoping that this would reduce the cost and increase the response rate) it gradually became clear that this approach was unfeasible and unattractive for our small research group.

A mailed approach was therefore chosen, and the ratio distribution and collection costs <u>versus</u> probable response rate was studied carefully. For the distribution, reduced bulk rates are available, but the return mail (collection) is an individual event for the postal system. Sole use of a business reply number as the only reply possibility was therefore not considered to be a useful option. We conducted a pilot study in 1985 among 1134 subjects to determine how the response rate would be affected by offering the respondents combinations of the following reply possibilities:
1. Provide your own stamp;
2. Use the business reply number;
3. Use a specified bank office as a local collection address.

The first possibility was part of every combination, and was indicated to be preferred by us. This pilot study showed that the addition of the bank option resulted in no worthwhile increase in response rates, considering the extra effort that would be required. The highest response rate (49.15) was reached when subjects could choose between a stamp and the business reply number. Since 85% of the respondents in this latter group in fact used a stamp, it appeared that the cohort study could be carried out within the limits of the budget. Consequently, the approach in which people could either use a stamp or the business reply number was used in the actual cohort study. In the pilot study, the effect on the response rate of requesting toenail clippings was also evaluated; this request resulted in an average decrease in the response rate of 2.8%.

The baseline survey was started in September 1986. At the same time, we started a nationwide publicity campaign on television, radio and newspapers to increase the response rate. The publicity was positive in general, although some critical remarks on the subject of privacy appeared in the press. One of the issues involved the use of the date of birth on the address label. This had been done deliberately in order to ascertain that the right person completed the questionnaire because, in mailed surveys, the problem exists that another person in the household (e.g. son or daughter with identical initials) may complete it. We had tested this system of address labels in the 1985 pilot study, at which time nobody commented on it. However, in the actual cohort study quite a number of people were upset about having their age marked on the envelope and refused to participate. This problem illustrates one of the choices an investigator has to make between, on the one hand, decreased response with more valid data and, on the other hand, a higher response rate with a number of questionnaires completed by the wrong persons.

At a later stage, a publicity campaign was used to remind people about the questionnaire and the deadline for completion. This appeared to be less successful than the campaign to introduce the study, since the "reminder" part of the text was omitted by the press. In addition to this free publicity we therefore put out advertisements in national and regional newspapers to convey our message that questionnaires were still welcome. (The use of personal reminders was prohibited by various participating municipalities.)

Response

Although we are still processing the returned material, it is possible to give preliminary resonse rates. These are based on numbers provided by the Dutch postal service (PTT) on the use of its business reply number and on the number of stamped questionnaires that we received.

The number of questionnaires returned during the first 5 weeks after the start of the study is depicted in Fig. 2, which also gives the daily relative contribution of business reply and stamp to the response. Unlike most mail surveys, the weekly response volume increased towards the fourth week (i.e. the last week before the deadline). This probably reflects the length of time and effort needed to complete the questionnaire. After 2 months, 121,309 questionnaires had been returned. Table 2 gives the response rate in more detail, as well as the proportion of stamp users. It shows that 67% of the respondents provided their own stamp, which is somewhat lower than indicated by the pilot study. However, an appreciable reduction in survey costs was accomplished in this way. No exact numbers on the proportion of respondents returning toenails can be given either at this moment, but a preliminary estimate of this equals 67% (i.e. 80 000 subjects).

The overall response rate of 35.6% is lower than we expected from the pilot study in 1985, which showed a response rate of 49%. Possible reasons for this decrease include: the use of a slightly longer questionnaire, the use of birth dates on the address label (over which there was a press upheaval), confusion with a national commercial survey which was held during the same period and which received a lot of negative publicity. The possibility, therefore, that the pilot population may not be completely representative of the final municipal sample will have to be evaluated.

Another form of representativeness, namely that of the respondents with regard to the initial municipal sample, will also be evaluated by comparing some of the exposure data with available national survey data. Because of the prospective nature of the study design it is unlikely, however, that selection bias will occur due to nonparticipation. After all, the selected subjects do not have the illness at the start of the study (apart from the initial prevalent cancer cases).

What is of more interest in this longitudinal study, however, is the heterogeneity of the determinants found in the remaining cohort, since comparisons will be made within the cohort.

Assuming equal response rates among men and women, as was the case in the pilot study, we estimated the number of incident cases that will originate from the cohort of approximately 121 000 individuals in the first 5 years of follow-up (Fig. 3), using national data on first hospital admissions and correcting for mortality (Central Bureau of Statistics, 1981a, 1981b, 1982). Approximately 300 stomach cancer, 400 colon cancer, 200 rectal cancer, 700 breast cancer and 1200 lung cancer cases are expected to arise from this cohort.

In the forthcoming statistical analyses, these cases will be compared to a sample of the cohort (the base) in a case-base approach. This "control" group will be selected immediately after identification of the cohort, by means of stratified random sampling. In Fig. 3 the size of this random sub-cohort is given as 3500, but a final decision on its size has not yet been taken. Detailed follow-up information on these individuals will be obtained so that the number of person-years accumulated by the cohort can be estimated. The first record linkage with PALGA and the Cancer Registry and subsequent statistical analyses will be started 3 years after the start of the study.

In an attempt to quantify the intra-individual variation in the determinants and to determine the stability of the dietary pattern, every year we will select different subsamples of 250 subjects from the control group for repeated applications of the questionnaire. Further studies among the cases are also being planned, but these have to await the approval of the ethical committees of PALGA and the Cancer Registries, because our current agreement with them does not allow us any further contact with linked cases.

REFERENCES

Central Bureau of Statistics (1981a) Maandstatistiek Bevolking en Volksgezondheid, 29, pp. 46-61.

Central Bureau of Statistics (1981b) Maandstatistiek Bevolking en Volksgezondheid, 29 (suppl), pp. 64-69.

Central Bureau of Statistics (1982) Maandstatistiek Bevolking en Volksgezondheid, 30, pp. 42-44.

Central Bureau of Statistics (1985) Statistical Yearbook. The Hague, Staatsuitgeverij.

Table 1. Size and origin of the potential participants

Origin	Men	Women	Total
Municipal sample	169 001	170 732	339 733
Vegetarians recruited	202	504	706
Total	169 203	171 236	340 439

Table 2. Response to survey according to reply category

Reply category	Response		
	Number	% of total	% of respondents
Stamp	81 596	23.97	67.26
Business reply number	39 713	11.67	32.74
Refused/address unknown	1 239	0.37	−
Deceased	149	0.04	−
No reply	217 742	63.96	−
Total	340 439		

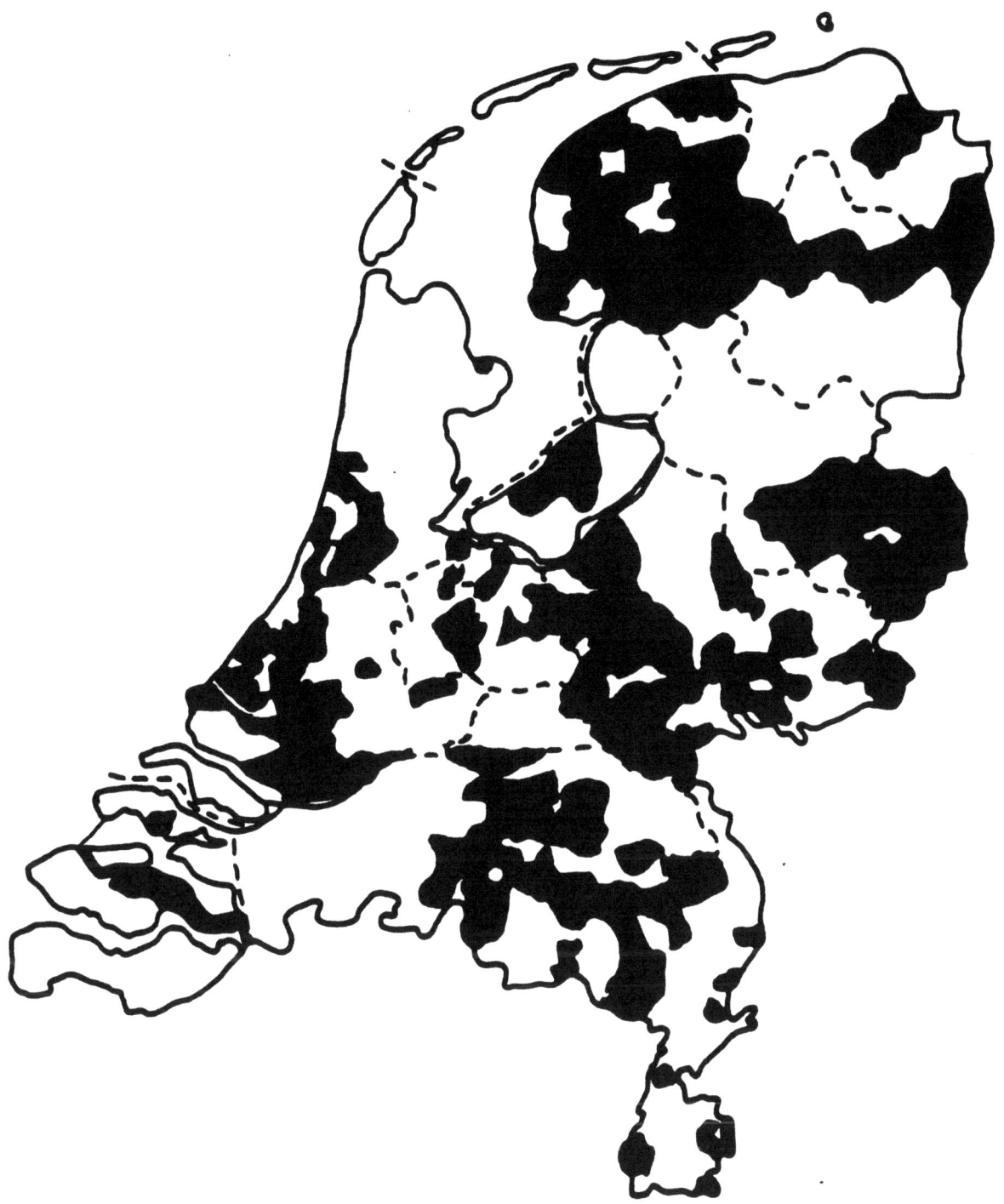

Figure 1. The location of the participating municipalities in the Netherlands.

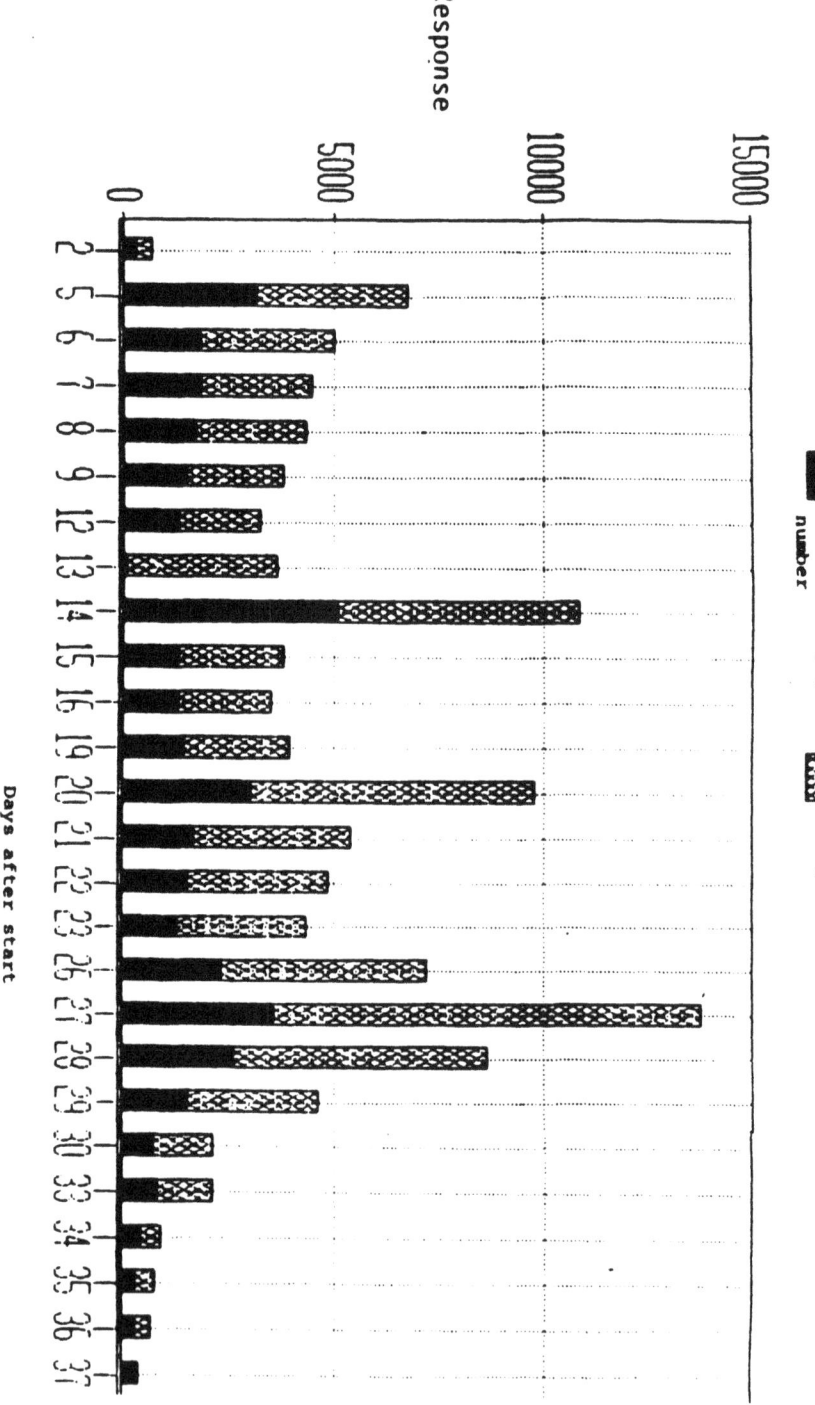

Figure 2. Daily response to survey during the first 5 weeks after the start.

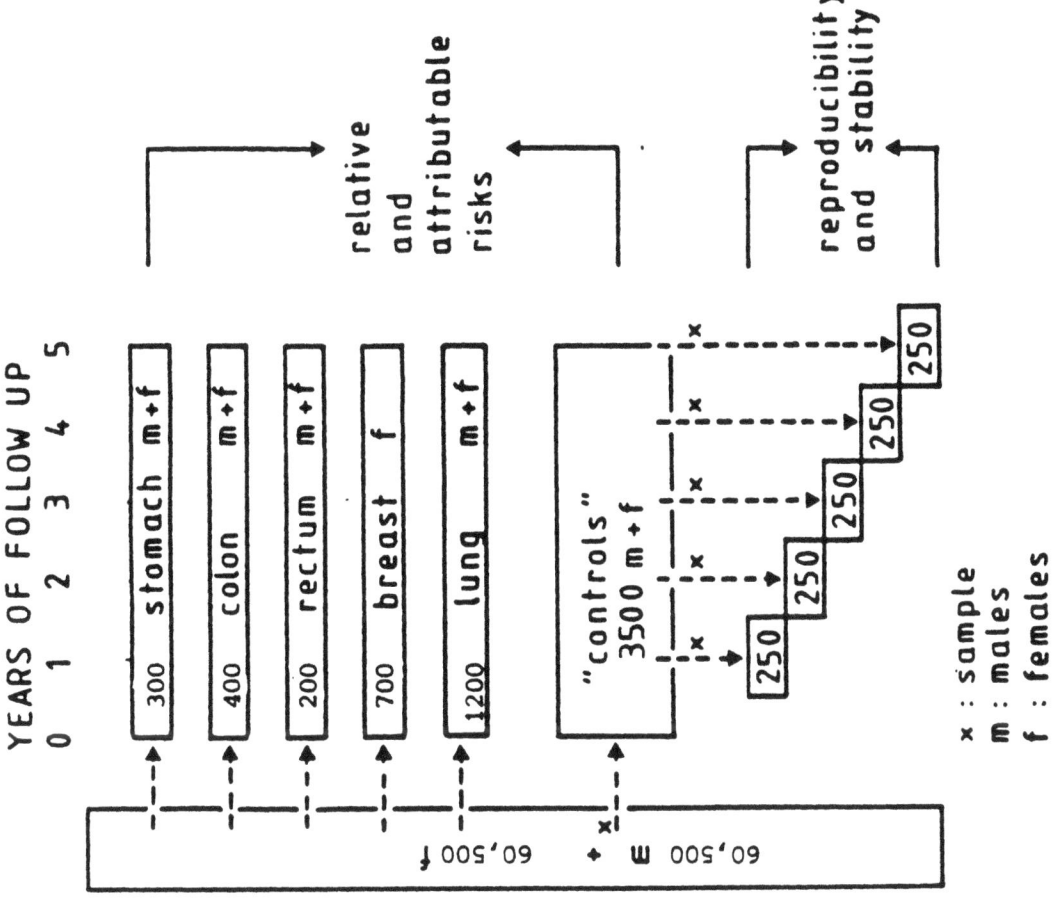

Figure 3. The design of the analysis of the Dutch cohort study on diet and cancer.

LOGISTICAL ASPECTS OF LONGITUDINAL STUDIES, WITH COLLECTION AND STORAGE OF BIOLOGICAL SAMPLES

H.J.A. Collette[1], A. Baanders-van Haleweijn[1], F. de Waard[2],

J.J. Rombach[1], P.A.H. van Noord[1]

[1] Preventicon Utrecht, Postbus 19006, 3501 DA Utrecht, The Netherlands

[2] Rijksinstitut voor de Volksgezondheid, Postbus 1, 3720 BA Bilthoven, The Netherlands

The DOM-Project (Diagnostisch Onderzoek Mammacarcinoom) is a population-based screening project to detect breast cancer at an early stage. The initial purpose was to combine it with a randomized nutritional intervention trial aimed a weight reduction. The rationale for this was the hypothesis that breast cancer would develop more slowly during and after weight reduction; if this were true, a longer interval between screenings would then be justified. However financial support was not obtained for such a large study. The project was therefore started as a non-randomized screening programme, with epidemiological research performed along various other lines. Various aspects of this research can be distinguished:

1. Is screening for breast cancer worth while? (Up to that time the HJP study was the only one of this kind.)
2. What will be the best way to perform a screening programme (length of interval, age limits, economic issues, etc.)?
3. What can be learned about the natural history and etiology of breast cancer?

From our experience of a population-based cervical screening programme, it was clear to us that this would be a long study for which we would need the assistance of clinicans and of local authorities. We therefore organized several meetings with pathologists, surgeons, general practitioners before the start of the project in order to ensure solid cooperation and valid registration. (For a screening project, 100% registration is a condition sine qua non.) A number of agreements were made and recorded with these physicians. In addition, a committee of counsellors was constituted to discuss problems and to advise us during the performance of the programme. The members of this committee came from various walks of life, i.e. local authorities, local health service, and also a "healthy woman" from a women's association.

We designed a questionnaire to be filled out by the participants themselves and checked by the paramedical assistants, and a form on which the results of the examination were to be noted. All data were to be coded (and initialed) according to strict rules, transferred to punch cards, and fed into the university computer. For example, one of the rules is the obligation to code every item, just to avoid mixing up negative answers and those which the respondent simply omitted.

In order to ensure good quality control, we trained the co-workers to fill out and code very precisely even when dealing with small, seemingly unimportant matters, because they cannot be held responsible for decisions concerning research aspects. Feedback by means of computer print-outs is another method of quality control.

As longitudinal studies continue over a long period of time and as, in the present study, intake was continuous and the study (and hence the number of people working on it) was large, it must be borne in mind that the chance of mistakes, misclassification and inaccuracy is multiplied (not to mention possible inter- and intra-observer variation). An extensive, properly written procedure manual has therefore to be drawn up. This is necessary not only for the co-workers but also for the person responsible for the study because with time it is easy to forget a great many points, most of them arbitrary.

In the Netherlands (thanks to Napoleon!) we are lucky to have population registries which make it possible to invite all people of, say, a given age, sex or residential area (with the permission and assistance of the above-mentioned local authorities). It is also possible to trace the number and identify of those women who did not attend. This is necessary when evaluating screening programmes in the short term.

As our programme was initially a research project and not a health service, we could afford to make a design well suited to epidemiological purposes. This means that only women who underwent the first examination were invited to participate in the second, and so on. An identification number was assigned to every woman giving the date of intake and a serial number of that day. All the information that we collect (and receive) after a referral for a biopsy about one woman will have the same number, including information about the course of the disease. The same holds for data from our breast cancer registry (e.g. false negatives) and causes of death. It is a considerable task to make sure that this is performed in a correct manner.

We started by inviting women born between 1911 and 1925 (i.e. 50-64 years old), and subsequently birth cohorts 1926-1931, 1932-1941 and 1942-1945 were invited. At the moment we are compelled by the Ministry of Health, which has been providing the funds since 1985, to use the latest population register of the city (the "WVC-programme"), so we have to link data from that register to our own data system when women are visiting our screening centre. Experiments on this are in progress. Table 1 gives the numbers of women participating and the repeat examinations.

When our programme was started there was interest in hormonal excretion in urine as a possible means of investigating whether it was possible to define a high-risk group for breast cancer that could be selected for screening. All women were therefore asked to bring along with them "night urine". As it was not possible to perform the laboratory tests on the same day, the samples were stored at $-20^{\circ}C$. As mentioned previously, they were all given an identification number.

After we had finished this sub-project, it was necessary to decide whether we should store these samples for a long period or not. As fund raising was going well at that time, we were able to start our bank of biological material with one or two urine samples from approximately 15,000 women, i.e. approximately 27,000 samples (one to two times 2,700 litres, i.e. around 6,000 pints). This has now been expanded up to 80,000 samples from 30,000 women. In addition we collected blood samples ($\pm$ 6,000) and toenails ($\pm$ 20,000).

Research on Other Diseases

Soon after the start of the DOM-Project, it became clear that it would be possible to collect data for research on other diseases in the same cohort. In the invitation letter for the first examination we explained that the respondents would participate in a research project. This means that there would be questions in the questionnaire for which the relation with breast cancer would not be clear to everyone. We promised that the confidentiality of the answers would be protected by our code of professional secrecy. Although we did not encounter any problems then, in subsequent screenings, when introducing research on other diseases, we mentioned that we were investigating other chronic diseases as well. By accepting this and visiting our centre, the participants gave informal rather than "informed consent" (although they did not sign).

In this manner our data base became rather extensive. The problems we met then were within our own group, because it can be very difficult to restrict oneself; we had to make scientific choices and refrain from spreading our resources too thinly over a wide area. The problem was to identify what subjects would be of interest in the (near) future. We had to make the difference between:
- what is desired,
- what is needed,
- what is available.

The attached synopsis (Table 2) shows the topics we have included. Some subjects have been merely touched upon while others are studied more or less in greater depth. Some are studied in all participants while others are only collected from specific birth cohorts or screening groups. As long as our screening programme is considered to be a research project, no problems are expected if some epidemiological research is added, and it is to be hoped that this research orientation remains if a nation-wide screening programme is to be organized.

From a logistic point of view we can divide our research on diseases other than breast cancer into several categories:

a) Collecting extra data and material during screening for a specific study.
b) Analysing the collected data from the point of view of a new, different hypothesis.
c) Linking the collected data with other already on-going registrations or with a registration particularly set up for a specific new study (for this we use the communication lines of the breast cancer screening programme).
d) Carrying out new laboratory tests on specific or randomized samples out of the biological material bank, linked with the data bank.

The method can be truly prospective, prospective in retrospect or it may be a cohort-nested case-control study. An example of a study of type d) is as follows:

Case-control study of endometrial cancer within a cohort

A population-based prospective study was started as a continuation of an earlier retrospective case-control study based on the association of endometrial cancer with specific risk factors, i.e. obesity, hypertension, decreased glucose tolerance and late menopause. At that time, it also appeared that these phenomena were accompanied by increased extra-ovarian production of oestrogens. The hypothesis was that these oestrogens were produced by the adrenal cortex. Continuous oestrogen production could explain the later onset of menopause, because the decreasing oestrogen production by the ovaries during the climacteric may be supplemented by adrenal oestrogens to such an extent that the cycles would continue for a further period of time.

The study encompassed more than 14 000 women (participants in the DOM-Project) who at the time of intake were aged between 50 and 65. This population was followed up over a period of 7.5 years. Apart from the above-mentioned risk factors, the study included the risk factors of total body size, age at first birth and parity. To quantify the endometrial cancer risk, we compared for each of the risk factors the observed numbers with the expected numbers as calculated by reference to data received from an external source. A total of 43 cases of endometrial cancer were found in the studied population.

The results of the study were the following. With regard to obesity, it was confirmed that the risk increased considerably with overweight. Height appeared to be a distinct factor, the risk for the tallest women being three times that for the shortest (a similar tendency was found earlier for breast cancer). Combining overweight and height, the correlation between endometrial cancer and body size was calculated (formula for body surface area derived by Gehan and George). The correlation between body size and risk of endometrial cancer appeared to be more pronounced than that for overweight. A lower risk was found for the following cases: lower age at first birth, more children, lower age at marriage and lower age at menopause. This is the result of a univariate analysis. Multivariate analyses show that the age at menopause was the most important independent risk factor, followed by the Quetelets overweight index and the number of children, in that order.

Finally it was possible (by analysing the urine samples collected many years earlier) to identify the biochemical background of certain of the variables by showing that, some time before endometrial cancer was diagnosed, the patients concerned had had a higher oestrogen secretion level than the control women who remained free of this disease during the study period.

Table 1. Number of women participating in the DOM-Project

Year	No. of first examinations (i.e. participants)	No. of repeat examinations[1]	Total
1975	5 327	-	5 327
1976	6 940	4 248	11 188
1977	5 372	6 974	12 346
1978	4 102	7 141	11 243
1979	1 770	9 036	10 806
1980	-	10 739	10 739
1981	7 978	744	8 722
1982	9 659	420	10 079
1983	5 104	5 904	11 008
1984	3 896	6 364	10 260
1985	4 423	4 823[2]	9 246
1986	955	10 140[2]	11 095
TOTAL	55 526	66 533	122 059

[1] Varies from 2 to 5 examinations per woman
[2] Including all participants in the "WVC programme", not yet linked with the original DOM-Project.

Table 2. Data collection in the DOM-Project

Items about which data are collected from all participants:

Identification: Name
    Address
    Date of birth
Health insurance
Marital status
Fertility: Number of children
    Age at first birth
    Contraceptive use
Menopause Date of last cycle
    Artificial or not
History of breast disease
Breast cancer in mother and/or sisters
Diet
Use of drugs
Anthropometry: Weight
    Height
Breast: Inspection
    Palpation
    Mammography
Breast cancer
Cause of death

Items about which data are collected in some birth cohorts or at a following screening examination (no specific order):

Osteoporosis	Epileptic insults
MI / CVA / TIA	Bowel habits
Famine history	Asthmatic diseases
T & A	Twins
Skin abnormalities	Breast feeding
Headache	Breast size
Food frequency items	BSE
Selenium intake	Blood pressure
Gallbladder & kidney stones	Anthropometry
Smoking habits	Laboratory: Urine
Drinking habits	Blood
Joint diseases	Nails

PROSPECTIVE STUDY OF HORMONES AND DIET IN THE ETIOLOGY OF BREAST CANCER
Synthesis of the project

F. Berrino[1], P. Pisani[1], P. Muti[1], P. Crosignani[1], S. Panico[2], M. Pierotti[1], G. Secreto[1], A. Totis[1], R. Fissi[1] & C. Mazzoleni[1]

[1] Istituto Nazionale Tumori, Milano, Italy

[2] Istituto di Medicina Interna e Malattie Dismetaboliche, 2a, Facolta' di Medicina Universita' di Napoli, Italy

The aim of our project is to clarify the role of sexual hormones in the etiology of breast cancer (B.C.), to ascertain and quantify the effect of dietary habits, and to study the relation between these two factors.

The choice of a prospective design, based on the recruitment of an ample cohort of initially healthy women, and of their epidemiological surveillance over a period of several years, derives firstly from the necessity to measure the exposure - hormonal profile and dietary intake - before the onset of the disease, secondly to assure that the exposure characteristics in women who eventually will develop breast cancer can be compared with a sample, representative of the cohort to which they belong.

STUDY DESIGN AND SIZE

a) **10.000 healthy women volunteers** residing in the province of Varese, and willing to be examined, complete questionnaires and supply blood and urine samples will be recruited. Only women who have not received hormone treatment recently nor had an oophorectomy, will be eligible for the study. Specimens are then collected according to strict standardized procedures.

b) Preparation of a **data bank** of controlled quality (but not codified) covering all factors (environmental, reproductive and constitutional) commonly recognised as of major importance in the etiology of B.C., and a **biological bank** where specimens are preserved at $-80^{\circ}C$.

A biological bank has both the economical advantage of carrying out biochemical tests only on those women who will develop B.C. and a small sample of those who will remain disease free, as well as the possibility to preserve material for testing hypotheses which at present are not clearly formulated, or for which there is no suitable laboratory technique.

c) **Follow-up** of the cohort through the Lombardy Cancer Registry, which has been operating in the Varese province since 1976, integrated with an *ad hoc* information system of participants moving from the Varese province.

135 incident cases of breast cancer are expected within the first ten years of follow-up. Biological specimens and anamnestic information previously collected will be analysed only for the cases, with an appropriate number of controls per case.

The study size allows a minimum of 80% probability of detecting a relative risk of 2 at a significant level of 1% when comparing the highest quartile with the three lower quartiles.

ETIOLOGICAL HYPOTHESES

A) Hormonal hypotheses

ORDET's basic hypothesis is the <u>ovarian androgens excess theory</u> devised by Professor Grattarola at the end of the 1960's. Other hormonal hypotheses concerning breast cancer are also considered plausible. However, as results from the various centres of research tend to be both complex and inconsistent, it is essential to carry out a study which considers several different physiological and pathological hypotheses simultaneously. We are also reliant on research into adrenal androgens, in oestrogenic profile, progesterone, SHBG, non SHBG bound steroids, and pituitary hormones.

This emphasizes the need to provide a <u>high number of aliquots</u>, and if necessary to refer to several different specialized laboratories at the moment of analysis. As refrigerator storage capacity is one of the major <u>economical bonds</u> of the project, the decision of the number and volume of aliquots had to be weighed against the planned number of participants.

The influence of the hormone profile on the development of B.C. may depend either on the haematic concentration, the periferic action, or the periferic metabolism of the same hormones. To obtain indicators of this periferical activity, it has been decided to observe several anthropometric variables, in order to define <u>body mass, fat distribution</u> (android or gynoid), <u>skin sebum production and hirsutism score</u>.

Apart from research into possible causal determinants of hormone levels, such as diet, menstrual and reproductive history, and familiarity of B.C., research is also made into the geopraphical origin, cultural background and sociological and psychological variables of each participant.

B) Dietary Hypotheses

It is of widespread opinion, sustained by many experimental and epidemiological studies, that a diet rich in <u>fats</u> especially animal fats, carries a higher risk of B.C.. Many epidemiological studies which have found this association however, show gross defects in either design or analysis.

It is probable that an association does exist, apparently not very strong, and therefore difficult to detect using simple dietary anamnesis techniques. It is also possible that diet is of more importance in the perimenarchial period. Furthermore, of the dietary studies so far carried out, hormonal variables have never been taken into account.

Epidemiological studies on certain <u>vitamins</u> and other <u>micro nutrients</u>, which have been found to be protective in experimental tests, have not as yet given us any consistent results.

More coherent results have been obtained on <u>alcohol</u> comsumption, even here though the association is rather modest and cannot be considered causal.

The aim of ORDET is to study the role of dietary habits <u>taking into account the levels of hormones</u>.

Dietary intake is investigated:

a) By determining the composition in fatty acids of the <u>red blood cell membranes</u>, which should reflect diet during the past few months.
b) By quantifying metallic elements in <u>nail</u> samples using the neutronic activation technique.
c) By determining various substances in <u>serum, plasma, urine and cytoplasm</u> (with particular interest in vitamins).
d) By <u>anamnestic investigation</u> into dietary intake. A dietary questionnaire has been specifically studied with the aim of quantifying the intake only of those foods which explain most of the variability of nutrients relevant to the study.

C) <u>Genetic hypotheses</u>

Studies on the familiarity of B.C. show serious methodological limits. The more reliable studies reveal that there are few families in which the risk is very high, while most of the familiar clusters could be explained from the high frequency of the disease. Presently, the identification and characterization of genic sequences possibly associated with disease, takes advantage from restriction fragment length polymorphism (RFLP) analysis. The association of specific RFLP (e.g. at protooncogene loci) with B.C. patients, may suggest a particular susceptibility of individuals to B.C.. Furthermore, the study of FRLP distribution in high risk families may lead to the identification of specific genetic markers segregating with the illness. Recently, RFLP analyses have shown somatic loss of heterozygosity in human B.C. cell DNA. Therefore, whenever possible, B.C. tissue samples will also be preserved at $-80°C$.

Another genetic indicator which will be studied, is the activity level of <u>glucose-6-phosphate dehyrogenase</u> in red blood cell cytoplasm. There is some evidence that the deficiency of this enzyme could be associated with lower risk of cancer. Genetic studies within ORDET will probably be made easier by the participation of a high number of women with a family history of B.C.

ORGANIZATION OF A BIOLOGICAL BANK

A 40 ml blood sample, 20 ml of which is treated with heparin, is used to prepare six 1.3 ml aliquots of <u>serum</u>, six 1.5 ml aliquots of <u>plasma</u>, 3 aliquots of <u>red blood cell membranes</u>, 3 aliquots of red blood cell <u>cytoplasm</u> and 3 aliquots of leucocytes for the preparation of <u>DNA</u>. Six 2 ml aliquots are prepared from a 12 hour urine collection (from 7.30 p.m. to 7.30 a.m.). A total of 27 aliquots of biological specimens per participant are subdivided in 3 freezers (9 aliquots per freezer).

Each freezer contains 640 containers of 81 compartments (9 rows of 9, i.e. 1 row per participant). Therefore each freezer contains specimens of 640 x 9 = 5760 participants.

At present there are 4 large $-80°C$ freezers (3 of which are in use, plus an empty spare one to be used in case of malfunction), 2 at Busto Arsizio hospital, near the main recruitment centre, and 2 at the Istituto dei Tumori in Milan, all provided with alarm systems and connected to a generator and to CO_2 cylinders. For maximum security against possible electricity blackouts, provision has been made to transfer a third of the aliquots in liquid nitrogen.

In order to permit a chromatographic determination of the sexual hormone profile in urine, which requires a sample of greater quantity per woman, a single aliquot of 50 ml (taken from the night urine) is stored in a freezer at -30°C.

A toenail sample will also be stored, for the determination of metal concentration, using neutronic activation techniques.

RECRUITMENT PROCEDURE

The main operating unit is at Busto Arsizio Breast Screening Centre. A second unit is located at Varese hospital. Both recruit women who have either voluntarily made an appointment for a check-up, or have been requested to attend a breast screening.

Women are briefly informed of the purpose of the project and asked if they would be willing to co-operate. Those accepting are subsequently registered and if eligible, an appointment is then made for a blood sample to be taken (as soon as possible in the case of women in menopause, or between the twentieth and twenty-fourth day of the menstrual cycle), between 8.00 a.m. and 9.00 a.m. on an empty stomach. The participants are then requested to complete an anamnestic questionnaire on their menstrual and reproductive history, and undergo brief psychometric tests.

An anthropometric visit is then carried out to register weight, height, height when seated, circumferences, skin folds, blood pressure, pulse rate, hirsutism score and sebum production.

Participants are then given an envelope containing an introductory letter, instructions and a dietary questionnaire (to be completed at home), and are provided with containers for the 12 hours urine collection and for toenail samples which they must bring with then on the day the blood sample is taken.

When the participant arrives for the appointment, the exact time the blood sample is taken is registered, blood pressure and pulse rate are once again measured, and another small aliquot of urine is taken.

Women who are in the menstrual or perimenstrual period, are given an appropriate from (to be returned by post) on which they indicate the first day of the following menstrual cycle and a calender for registering menstrual cycle dates for the subsequent 6 months.

PRELIMINARY STUDIES

Each decision made regarding the planning of ORDET, is based on feasibility studies and practical tests. The most important studies carried out, or in progress, are the following:

1) Validity of the participants classification in terms of the urine levels of certain hormones measured in the 12 hour night urine sample as compared to the 24 hour urine sample.
2) Circadian variation of serum concentration of sexual hormones.
3) Inter-individual variability of serum and urine concentration of certain hormones.
4) Repeatability of the anthropometric measurements.
5) Repeatability of certain sections of the anamnestic questionnaire.
6) Repeatability of the dietary questionnaire and its validity compared to more sophisticated techniques of dietetic surveys.
7) Validity of the composition of fatty acids of the red blood cell membranes (compared to a biopsy of adipose tissue) as a nutritional indicator.
8) Validity of the determination of metallic elements in nail samples as a nutritional indicator.
9) Control of the reservation over time of biological specimens.

IDEAS FOR A POSSIBLE PROSPECTIVE STUDY ON SUBJECTS BELONGING TO A HEALTH INSURANCE PLAN IN PARIS

F. Clavel, F. Doyon, R. Flamant

I.N.S.E.R.M. U 287, Institut Gustave Roussy, Villejuif, France

Breast cancer and cancer of the large intestine (colon and rectum) are very common. In France, breast cancer is the most frequent among females, whereas colorectal cancer is the most frequent among people of both sexes consered together. Breast and right-colon are (together with gall-bladder) the sole sites of cancer which cause more deaths among females than among males.

We have calculated the international correlation between breast or intestinal cancer and different cancer sites and in 33 selected countries in the world have found that there is a very high correlation ($r = 0.81$) between breast and intestinal cancer. So it may be hypothesised that these cancers share some risk factors, of hormonal origin. To test this hypothesis, a large cohort study focused on cancer of the breast and of the large intestine has been planned. This study would be undertaken in France on 10 000 female volunteers belonging to a Health Insurance Plan.

The study we plan to conduct will be focused on (i) the relation between precursors of disease and breast cancer, (ii) the study of the risk factors for colon cancer, mainly hormonal factors, and (iii) the genetic epidemiology of cancer of the breast and of the large intestine. The first point is to study the relationship between benign breast disease and breast cancer. In the literature, 17 observational studies have appeared - two case-control studies and 15 cohort studies - for which the follow-up period ranges from 2.5 to 30 years. Some studied all women who had biopsy-defined benign breast disease, some restricted the study to certain histological types of lesions, and others only considered scores of cytologic atypia.

It would appear from previous studies that (a) a history of biopsy-defined benign breast disease increases the risk of breast cancer, and (b) the risk is increased for the more hyperplastic or epithelial proliferative forms of benign disease. However, can these general impressions be considered as real evidence? Firstly, with regard to point (a), in the case-control studies it can be seen that there is possible recall bias when women with breast cancer are interviewed on their personal histories; in cohort studies, there is a possible selection bias because women at high risk of breast cancer may be biopsied more often than others and also because women with biopsy-defined benign breast disease may have more frequent breast examinations that lead to the discovery of breast cancer. With regard to point (b), the more hyperplastic or epithelial proliferative forms of benign breast disease could be considered to have the same etiology as breast cancer if the risk factors are the same. This does not appear to have been demonstrated yet, although some studies on this topic are on-going, but not yet published.

Our study would provide some answers to these unresolved questions by analyzing the risk of breast cancer for women who have had a benign breast disease, by histopathological sub-type, and by studying risk factors for non-biopsied benign breast disease, and biopsied breast disease by different histopathological sub-types. In our study, benign breast disease would be defined from mammography, and by reference to the initial mammography some (of course) being ascertained by biopsy.

The second aim of our study is to examine the genetic epidemiology of breast and colon cancer. Up to now we know that there is consistent epidemiological evidence of a relationship between a family history of breast cancer and further occurrence of breast cancer. This evidence is less conclusive for colorectal cancer. Different reasons were proposed for such familial aggregations. The first one is chance, since these cancers are common, the second is that the same risk factors may be present among the different members of the family, and the third reason might be genetic susceptibility which seems to be controlled by a dominant autosomal gene. However, because of different biases or because of methodological inadequacies, this assumption requires further consideration.

We therefore plan a prospective study to collect new data on the prevalence in the family of cancer of any site, and of the main breast cancer risk factors. Our data would be reliable because it should not be affected by recall bias. Our intention is to apply segregation analysis to study the genetic susceptibility to breast cancer and to colorectal cancer and also to separate genetic from environmental risk factors for breast cancer, and to search for links between colon and breast cancer.

In the literature there are several studies on the possible relation between hormonal factors and colon cancer, but the results are still inconclusive.

Our study will be a cohort study on 10 000 women whom we initially plan to follow-up for ten years. The women will be teachers belonging to a Health Insurance Plan. They should volunteer to participate, i.e. to agree to fill in the yearly follow-up questionnaire, to undergo an initial mammography, and to have a blood specimen taken. They should be aged 40 to 65 and live in the Paris metropolitan area, and should not, of course, have any personal history of breast or colorectal cancer.

The initial check-up will consist of a questionnaire of general and genetic epidemiology, a mammography, and the taking of a blood specimen in order to set up a serum and a lymphocyte bank. The follow-up of our volunteers should be fairly easy because the Health Insurance Plan routinely records any change of address, all deaths occurring and all visits to doctors (the name of the doctor and the purpose of the visit). Any occurrence of cancer is also registered. With regard to hospitalization, only the name of the hospital is recorded, but we plan to look at the hospitals' files in order to learn the purpose of the hospitalization.

During the period of ten years of follow-up, we expect around 200 cases of breast cancer and around 50 colon cancer cases.

This study is still at the planning stage, and will be started as soon as a number of logistic problems have been solved.

OVERVIEW OF PROSPECTIVE STUDIES ON DIET, CANCER AND CARDIOVASCULAR DISEASES IN FINLAND

P. Pietinen, J. Virtamo & J.K. Huttunen

National Public Health Institute, 166 Mannerheimintie, 00280 Helsinki, Finland

BETA-CAROTENE, ALPHA-TOCOPHEROL LUNG CANCER INTERVENTION TRIAL

The US-Finland Studies of Nutrition and Cancer are a collaborative project conducted by the National Public Health Institute of Finland and the Division of Cancer Prevention and Control of the US National Cancer Institute. The other institutes involved are the Department of Food Chemistry and Technology, the Department of Nutrition (both in the University of Helsinki), the Social Insurance Institute and the Finnish Cancer Registry. While several aspects of the role of diet in cancer are being investigated in the project, the largest enterprise is a beta-carotene, alpha-tocopherol lung cancer intervention trial (Huttunen, 1985; Heinonen et al., 1987).

The primary objective of the trial is to evaluate the effectiveness of beta-carotene and alpha-tocopherol in preventing lung cancer in high risk smoking men aged between 50 and 69. Secondary objectives are: (a) to study the effect of beta-carotene and alpha-tocopherol supplementation on the incidence of cancer at other sites, and (b) to assess the association between the baseline intake of various nutrients and the risk of subsequent cancer. A study to evaluate the appropriateness of the case-control approach in diet and cancer studies is also nested in the trial (see below). The trial is a randomized double-blind, placebo-controlled experiment with a full two-factorial design. It involves four primary intervention groups: beta-carotene (20 mg), alpha-tocopherol (50 mg), beta-carotene and alpha-tocopherol (20 and 50 mg) and placebo, given in one capsule a day. This design will enable separation of the main effects of beta-carotene and alpha-tocopherol, and allow analysis of interactions, if any. About 20 000 men, aged between 50 and 69 and smoking at least five cigarettes a day, are recruited.

The trial participants are recruited from south and south-west Finland. The whole male population of this area in the age range 50 to 69 is approached by a postal questionnaire enquiring about smoking and willingness to participate. The postal survey is carried out in seven successive subsamples. The men smoking currently at least five cigarettes per day and willing to participate are invited to an initial examination. This includes smoking and occupational histories, dietary assessment, blood pressure, height, weight, and visual acuity measurements, chest X-ray and blood and toenail sampling. Lung cancer found in chest X-ray leads to exclusion. Other exclusion criteria are previous malignancy other than nonmelanoma skin or carcinoma-in-situ, severe angina on effort, chronic renal insufficiency, liver cirrhosis, alcoholism, anticoagulant therapy, and regular use of beta-carotene, vitamin A or E. Written informed consent is obtained from each eligible subject.

The participants are enrolled over a period of two years in 1985-1987. After recruitment the participants make a follow-up visit three times a year, i.e. every four to five months. The follow-up includes smoking and disease histories and symptom monitoring. At the visit the unused capsules are counted and a new capsule package is given. The intervention will last five to seven years and will end for every participant in spring 1992.

Occurrence of lung cancer during the latter four to six intervention years will be the primary end point. Cancers observed during the first trial year will be excluded from analysis since they probably evolved prior to the beginning of the intervention. The lung and other cancers will be verified by the Finnish Cancer Registry.

As the intervention agents used in the trial are vitamins or provitamins commonly found in normal diets, it is necessary to monitor dietary intake of these compounds and other potentially important nutrients. This will be accomplished through the use of two dietary survey instruments, a self-administered food use questionnaire, which includes questions on the usual frequency and portion size of over 200 food items, and a short food frequency questionnaire collecting frequency information only for those food items which are main sources of vitamins A (including carotenes), C and E, selenium, dietary fats and fibre. The former questionnaire is completed before randomization and the latter at the beginning of and once during the trial.

At the baseline cardiovascular and respiratory symptoms are also registered, and these inquiries are repeated annually. During the follow-up visits, any medical appointments and the reasons for them are recorded. Some of the diagnoses such as myocardial infarction and stroke are verified from hospital case reports. Thus this trial also offers an opportunity to study the association between diet and non-cancer diseases such as cardiovascular and respiratory diseases.

Case-control validity evaluation study

The validity of the case-control approach in studies on diet and cancer has not been fully evaluated. Tumour growth or awareness of the potentially fatal disease may influence dietary intake and metabolism of nutrients, or assessment of dietary intake. The intervention trial described above gives an opportunity to evaluate whether the possible differences in blood chemistry and dietary intake between cancer cases and controls occurred already years before the clinical cancer or whether they have developed recently.

During the last four to six years of the trial, approximately 600 lung cancer cases and 600 other cancer cases will be diagnosed among the participants. All the cases will be requested to fill in once again the self-administered food use questionnaire at home and to visit the local study centres as soon as possible after the discovery of cancer. Blood samples and toenails will be taken as at the initial examination. Throughout every year, 800 persons without known cancer will be randomly selected from the trial participants to serve as controls. These subjects will be send a food use questionnaire to be completed at home and returned at the next follow-up visit, when also blood and toenail samples will be collected.

For each case and each control, both baseline and follow-up case-control sera and questionnaire will be analysed for variables of interest, among others carotenes, retinol, tocopherols, and selenium. Two types of analyses will be conducted. First, the differences in pre- and post-diagnosis values will be examined in cases by site of cancer. Parallel analyses will be performed in the control group. Second, the difference between the means of case and control groups will be studied. Various independent factors influencing the dependent variable will be controlled.

Linkage of the nutrient data of the Social Insurance Institute with the cancer incidence data

In connection with a large population survey, the Social Insurance Institute of Finland collected blood samples from about 50 000 individuals between 1966 and 1972. These samples have been stored frozen at -20°C. Based on the social security number, Hakama et al. (1984) have linked the data from the serum bank with those from the Finnish Cancer Registry, and found 860 cancer cases. Two controls matched for sex, age and follow-up have been selected for each case. Tocopherol, beta-carotene, retinol and retinol binding protein will be analysed.

A dietary history interview was carried out in a random subsample of this population (5 224 men and 4 577 women). As a part of the US-Finland Studies of Nutrition and Cancer, this data will be linked with the data in the Finnish Cancer Registry. The number of cancer cases in this subsample by the end of 1986 will allow analyses on the association between the intake of various dietary components and the incidence of total cancer in both sexes, and the incidence of lung cancer in males and breast cancer in females.

CASE-CONTROL STUDIES BASED ON DATA COLLECTED IN EASTERN FINLAND

The data collected in the baseline survey of the North Karelia project in 1972 as well as in the terminal survey of the project in 1977 have been used prospectively. Both surveys comprised a random 6.7% sample of the population aged 25-59 (in 1977) or 30-64 (in 1977) living in two provinces of eastern Finland: North Karelia and Kuopio. Altogether about 10 000 people were examined in 1972 and about 12 000 in 1977.

A case-control study was conducted with data based on a seven-year follow-up of the population sample of 1972 to investigate the association between serum selenium and risk of death from acute coronary heart disease (CHD) as well as risk of fatal and non-fatal myocardial infarction (MI) (Salonen et al., 1982). A serum selenium concentration of less than 45 mg/litre was associated with an adjusted relative risk of CHD death of 1.9, and a relative risk of fatal and non-fatal MI of 2.1. Another matched-pair analysis was conducted with data based on a six-year follow-up of the same population sample to study the association between serum selenium and the risk of cancer (Salonen et al., 1984). A serum selenium concentration of less than 45 mg/litre was associated with a relative risk of cancer of 3.1. These data support the hypothesis that selenium deficiency increases the risk of CHD and certain cancers in middle-aged persons.

The independence and joint associations of serum selenium and vitamins A and E concentrations with the risk of death from cancer have also been studied in a case-control analysis of the four-year follow-up data from the 1977 survey (Salonen et al., 1985). The adjusted risk of fatal cancer was 5.8-fold among subjects in the lowest tertile of selenium concentrations compared with those with higher values. Subjects with both low selenium and low alpha-tocopherol concentrations in serum had an 11.4-fold adjusted risk. These data suggest that dietary selenium deficiency is associated with an increased risk of fatal cancer, that low vitamin E intake may enhance this effect, and that decreased vitamin or provitamin A intake contributes to the risk of lung cancer among smoking men with a low selenium intake.

These prospective studies based on both 1972 and 1977 survey data are still on-going, and new analyses based on longer follow-up periods will be conducted in the future.

KUOPIO ISCHAEMIC HEART DISEASE RISK FACTOR STUDY (KIHD)

The purpose of the Kuopio Ischaemic Heart Disease Risk Factor Study is to investigate the association of the course of life, physical activity, diet, smoking, social network participation and support, and personality with the risk of ischaemic heart disease (IHD) and with the progression of arteriosclerosis, and the underlying biological mechanisms. The study design comprises prospective follow-up of a total sample of approximately 1 200 men aged 54 and 1 800 men aged 50 from eastern Finland, the area with the highest recorded IHD incidence and mortality. Ultrasonography of carotid and peripheral arteries of the lower extremities and risk factor measurements are repeated after three years for surviving men who were 50 years old at entry. The risk factor measurements consist of interviews and self-administered questionnaires including 12-month and 7-day leisure time and occupational physical activity recalls, 24-hour physical activity recording, four-day supervised food recording, maximal exercise tolerance test with computerized ECG and direct breath-by-breath respiratory gas analysis, ambulatory 24-hour Holter-recording (for 50 year olds), and a comprehensive set of chemical and haematological tests from blood and urine. Special emphasis is on trace elements and vitamins, coagulation factors, thrombocyte aggregability, prostaglandins, catecholamines, serum lipids and apoproteins, and immunoglobulins.

The study is conducted jointly by the Kuopio University Research Institute of Public Health and Department of Community Health, Kuopio Research Institute of Exercise Medicien, and the National Public Health Institute, Helsinki. The principal investigator is Professor Jukka T. Salonen, University of Kuopio and the Co-PI Dr Rainer Rauramaa. The initial survey on risk factors is being carried out between 1984 and 1989. Gathering data on deaths and other disease events will be completed by the end of 1993.

REFERENCES

Hakama, M., Aaran, R.M., Aromaa, A. et al. (1984) Linkage of the data on biological sample bank of blood and Cancer Registry in Finland. Abstract. Bergen, Norway, Third Nordic Meeting on Nutrition

Heinonen, O.P., Virtamo, J., Albanes, D. et al. (1987) Beta-carotene, alpha-tocopherol lung cancer intervention trial in Finland. Helsinki, XI IEA Meeting

Huttunen, J.K. (1985) Studies on diet, nutrition and cancer in Finland. In: Joossens, J.V., Hill, M. & Geboers, J., eds, Diet and Human Carcinogenesis, Amsterdam, Elsevier, pp. 199-206

Salonen, J.T., Alfthan, G., Huttunen, J.H., Pikkarainen, J. & Puska, P. (1982) Association between cardiovascular death and myocardial infarction and serum selenium in a matched-pair longitudinal study. Lancet, ii, 175-179

Salonen, J.T., Alfthan, G., Huttunen, J.K. & Puska, P. (1984) Association between serum selenium and the risk of cancer. Am. J. Epidemiol., 120,, 342-439

Salonen, J.T., Salonen, R., Lappetelainen, R., Maenpaa, P.H., Alfthan, G. & Puska, P. (1985) Risk of cancer in relation to serum concentrations of selenium and vitamins A and E: matched case-control analysis of prospective data. Br. Med. J., 290, 417-420

CONTRIBUTION OF POPULATION SCREENING PROGRAMMES FOR THE RECRUITMENT OF SUBJECTS TO BE FOLLOWED PROSPECTIVELY

F. Lindgärde

Department of Medicine, University of Lund, Malmö General Hospital, 214 01 Malmö, Sweden

Malmo is a town in the south of Sweden with a population of about 230,000. It has just one hospital which is part of the University of Lund. The Department of Preventive Medicine, an integral part of the Department of Medicine, is located in an apartment house just outside the hospital area. It has been in operation since 1975, and its role is the detection of risk factors for non-infectious diseases, particularly those associated with cardiosclerosis and borderline alcoholism.

The invited subject meets a nurse who peforms the examination, takes blood samples and a short oral medical history. Since we are particularly interested in the development of diabetes mellitus type II, we perform an oral glucose tolerance test (OGTT). During the OGTT the subject has to answer about 200 questions, and the answer "yes", "no" or "don't know" is stored in the computer. It can be analysed immediately together with the blood test results. We have an attendance rate of about 75% for both sexes (Table 1). In about 30% of those who are examined, we have to check one or several values, and after that we are informed if the result of the medical examination has been satisfactory, or if it is necessary to refer the subject to different outpatient clinics or to the Department of Medicine or other clinics at the hospital. In borderline cases, a new examination takes place one, two or five years later.

As mentioned above, we have been particularly interested in evaluating our preventive efforts with respect to cardiovascular and alcohol-related diseases.

The cut-off levels that we use for intervention purposes are rather high, and this is a consequence of our lack of capacity to take care of all those subjects in whom we detect borderline disease. For instance a diastolic blood pressure level at or above 105 mm Hg is usually considered too high. However, such an individual is re-examined one year later.

Table 2 indicates that there is an unfavourable metabolic profile regarding males in comparison to the female population, and in my opinion this may partly explain why Swedish women have a life expectancy of 79.5 years compared to 73 for men. This difference was not apparent about 70 years ago, and it has been hypothesized that this may be a result of urbanization. Pulmonary function (FEV %) is more disturbed in males as a result of the higher frequency of smoking. The difference in diastolic blood pressure levels is a consequence of the fact that men are not as well treated as women with respect to blood pressure (Table 3). The prevalence of hypertension is similar in both sexes - 8.5% and 10.2%, respectively.

I have been involved in a diabetes cohort study in which we have followed males for about eight years with respect to glucose tolerance. As shown in Table 1, we invited 9,000 males aged 47 to 49 (mean age 48), and about 7,000 responded to the invitation; the non-respondent rate was about 25%. We performed an oral glucose tolerance test in all individuals who had

had no diagnosis of diabetes mellitus. In about 6% of this population, i.e. about 400 individuals, impaired glucose tolerance (IGT) according to WHO criteria was diagnosed. About six years after the first examination we reinvited the total cohort, and evaluated glucose tolerance again. The prevalence of diabetes in the cohort was 4%. During that period we were interested in following up whether the group identified as having IGT developed diabetes or not. In spite of non-pharmacological treatment, dietary advice and encouragement to increase physical fitness, 14% of the IGT group developed diabetes mellitus compared to 2% in the group with quite normal glucose tolerance.

The second aim of our study was to see if it was possible to prevent cardiovascular disease incidence in that particular group, i.e. those with IGT. We know from other studies, for instance the Whitehead study and the Paris prospective study that an increased number of individuals in the IGT group suffer myocardial infarction and strokes. We also tried to evaluate if diet had anything to do with the development of diabetes, and very briefly I can say that the development of diabetes seems to be inversely related to fibre intake, and change in bodyweight seems to be positively related to fat intake. Mortality in the different glucose tolerance groups has been analysed. The IGT Group, in which we have been particularly interested, seems to have the same mortality as the total group, which may indicate that the intervention programme has been successful in spite of the increased prevalence of diabetes in this group.

With regard to the specific issues that we are discussing at this meeting, we have performed a study together with the Swedish Medical Research Council, and our hosts for this meeting, Drs Riboli and Saracci. The aim of our study was to collect health data in a representative group of people living in Malmö, aged between 55 and 69, and to assess different dietary methods during a period of one year (Dr Callmer in this Report). I have some preliminary data here, that is perhaps of some interest.

In 1984 we invited 879 individuals aged between 50 and 69, representing 1% of the population. The attendance rate was 66.8%. During the medical examination we referred about 10% of this study group to other departments; 559 subjects agreed to take part in the dietary assessment. The reason for combining these two surveys was of course that we expected to be able to increase the number of participants in the dietary study if we offered a free medical health examination at the same time. However, it turned out that we were not able to reach the same attendance rate as for the normal health screening procedure that has been operating in Malmö for the last ten years.

We invited the 559 subjects again one year later. At that time we performed the medical examinations in the morning after the subjects had fasted for 12 hours. Of those who started the study one year earlier, 89% attended the Institute for a health examination, following which we had to refer about 8% to various outpatient clinics for a further check-up due to conditions such as diabetes, uncontrolled hypertension, anaemia, mental problems, etc.

Table 3 shows some clinical data which indicate that there is a substantial increase in cardiovascular diseases in this age group compared to the 48 year old age group. I want to point out from my position as a clinician that it is very important, when we discuss the reliability of different dietary measurements, that we take into consideration that in a group with a mean age of 59.5, 21-23% of that population are under treatment or have blood pressure values that are considered to be abnormal. This information is very important because those biochemical markers in blood and urine that we want to measure as markers for dietary intake of the nutritional status obviously might be changed by these different diseases in combination with medication.

Since, for various reasons, we were interested in evaluating the prevalence and the incidence of constant pain in joints and skeletal muscle, we asked a rheumatologist to examine all the participants who attended the first medical check-up in 1984, and he examined 99% of them. We tried to evaluate by means of letters, telephone calls and hospital records the prevalence in the non-respondent group. The "panorama" of these diagnoses is illustrated in Table 4. Group 1 is the respondents, and group 2 the non-respondents. We find very few people with rheumatoid arthritis. However, as one might expect, osteoarthritis was the dominant diagnosis. In the respondent group 24% complained of constant pain for more than five weeks, and of course they had taken medication during that period. In my opinion, this is another valuable piece of information, i.e. that normal people in this age group have such a high prevalence of constant pain localized in muscles, tendons and arteries. We call them a healthy group, but they do not consider themselves to be healthy. In contrast to other diagnoses, we found a surprisingly low prevalence of pain in the non-respondent group, and we have no valid explanation for this. This finding is in contrast to other diagnoses that we have examined with respect to cardiovascular disease, alcoholism and diabetes that are higher in the non-respondent group.

Table 1. Numbers of men and women examined at the age of 48 in the Malmö Cohort Study

	Men (5 age cohorts)	Women (1 age cohort)
Invited	9033	1288
Respondents	6975	951
% responding	77.2%	73.8%

Table 2. Percentages of subjects above cut-off levels at the age of 48

		Women	Men
Diastolic blood pressure 10	$\geq$ 105 mm	1.6%	8.4%
Cholesterol	$\geq$ 7.7 mmol/l	2.7%	4.3%
Triglycerides	$\geq$ 2.5 mmol/l	2.3%	11.5%
GT (gammaglutamyl-transferase)	$\geq$ 1.38 cal/l	3.0%	10.2%
Fasting blood glucose	$\geq$ 5.8 mmol/l	6.0%	7.1%
FEV % 1.0 sec	< 70%	5.7%	17.1%

Table 3. Prevalence of cardiovascular diseases in two age groups (50-69[a] and 48)

	Women		Men	
	Age 50-69	Age 48	Age 50-69	Age 48
Hospitalized for myocardial infarction	1.7%	0.1%	7.2%	1.1%
Angina pectoris	5.8%	1.2%	8.9%	1.8%
Treatment for hypertension	16.9%	7.2	16.4%	5.2%
Newly detected hypertension, 1984	2.1%	-	4.4%	-
Newly detected hypertension, 1985	2.4%	-	2.4%	-
Prevalence of hypertension	21.4%	8.5%	23.2%	10.2%

[a]Mean age 59.5

Table 4. Prevalence of pain in joints and skeletal muscle

	I (%)	II (%)
Rheumatoid arthritis	0.8	0.6
Other chronic arthritis	1.1	0.9
Osteoarthritis	13.2	6.8
Unspecified arthralgias	5.2	3.7
Fibrositis	1.5	0.9
Shoulder pain	7.3	4.6
Low back pain	7.8	
Neck pain	7.3	

PLANS FOR A PROSPECTIVE STUDY ON DIET AND CANCER IN DENMARK

Marianne Ewertz

Danish Cancer Registry, 66 Landskronagade, 2100 Copenhagen Ø, Denmark

It has been estimated that 10-70% of all cancers in the United States may be related to diet. It is justified to assume that a similar proportion is attributable to diet in Denmark, where up to 80% of all cancers occur at sites for which dietary components, nutrients or nutritional status have been implicated as possible risk factors (Figs. 1a and 1b). Most of the current evidence of an association between diet and cancer is based on international correlations and the results of case-control studies. While the former do not necessarily reflect causality, case-control studies may be biased by the presence of the malignant disease and difficulties in recalling dietary habits of the past. It is therefore proposed that a large prospective cohort study be conducted to examine the association in individuals between specific dietary components, foods or nutrients - alone or in combination - and the risk of cancer of specific sites.

A number of specific hypotheses will be tested from existing knowledge of diet and various types of cancer, for example:

- Does a high intake of fat increase the risk of cancers of the colon and rectum?

A further objective is to create a data bank of information on dietary factors, personal habits and to have biological samples available to test future hypotheses on cancer risk.

The study population will consist of a random sample of 63 500 persons aged between 40 and 54, drawn from the Central Population Register. A complete sampling frame exists by virtue of the personal ID-numbers which have been issued to all persons living in and entering the country (by birth or immigration) since 1968. It can be estimated that about 1000 persons in the population will have a cancer, i.e. prevalent cases. They will be excluded from the study cohort by record linkage to the cancer registry. Information on usual adult diet and known important risk factors for cancer, such as smoking and reproductive history, will be obtained by a combined self-administered/ interviewer-checked questionnaire. Anthropological measurements (height, weight, skinfold thickness will be made, and biological samples (blood, urine, hair, nails) collected for storage and later analysis. Biological sampling should be repeated if possible, and follow-up questionnaires will be mailed every 3 years to participants to assess dietary changes. The study population will be followed to record cases of cancer, death and emigration by linkage to the Cancer Registry and the Central Population Register. Follow-up for other diseases will be done by record linkage with other disease registries. With the combined use of these registries, an almost complete follow-up is envisaged, i.e. close to 100% of enrolled persons.

With an anticipated response rate of 80%, dietary data will be available from approximately 50 000 men and women. Based on current cancer rates, it can be estimated that some 3 900 cancer cases will develop within 10 years; the expected numbers and site distribution appear in Table 1. After an initial planning and pilot phase of 18 months, the baseline data collection will take one year. The cohort will be followed for at least 10 years. Contact has been made with colleagues in other Nordic countries for the establishment of parallel studies in Finland, Norway, Sweden and Iceland, which could eventually lead to a cohort comprising several hundred thousand persons for joint analysis.

Table 1. Number and site distribution of cancers expected in the study cohort (25 000 men and 25 000 women) after 1, 5 and 10 years of follow-up

Sex	Site	Expected number of cancers developed after:		
		1 year	5 years	10 years
Men	All sites	70	602	1 945
	Lung	10	113	436
	Colon-rectum	7	65	210
	Bladder	5	48	155
	Melanoma	3	30	97
Women	All sites	112	775	1 938
	Breast	36	217	465
	Cervix uteri	10	70	174
	Corpus uteri	6	39	97
	Lung	8	54	135
	Colon-rectum	6	39	97
	Melanoma	6	39	97

Cancer in Denmark 1981-1982

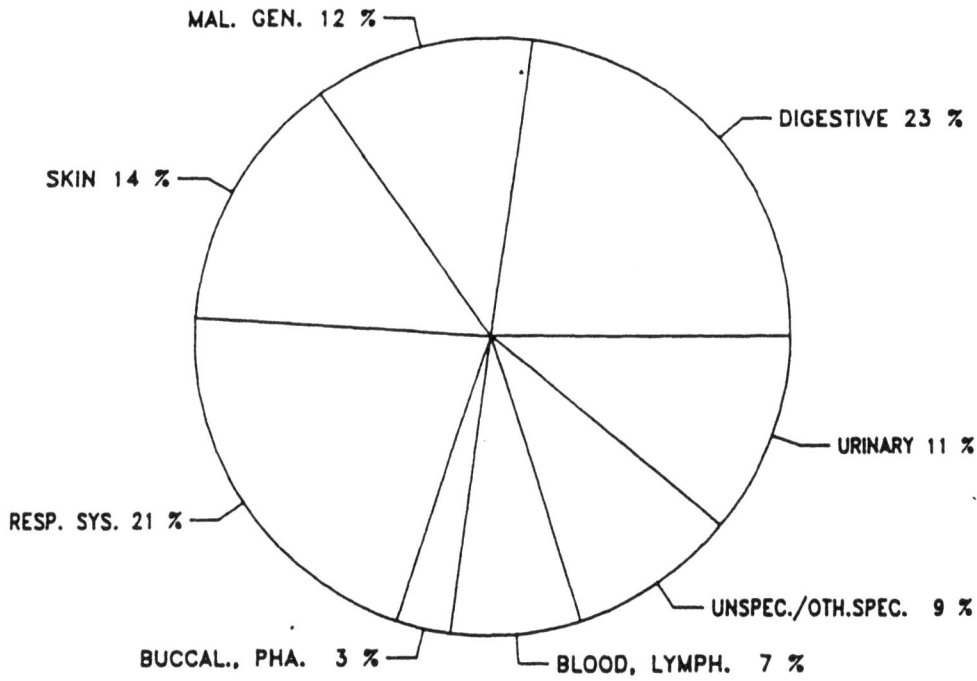

Fig. 1a: Proportional distribution of the age standardized incidence rates (World population) on different organs. Males, 1982.

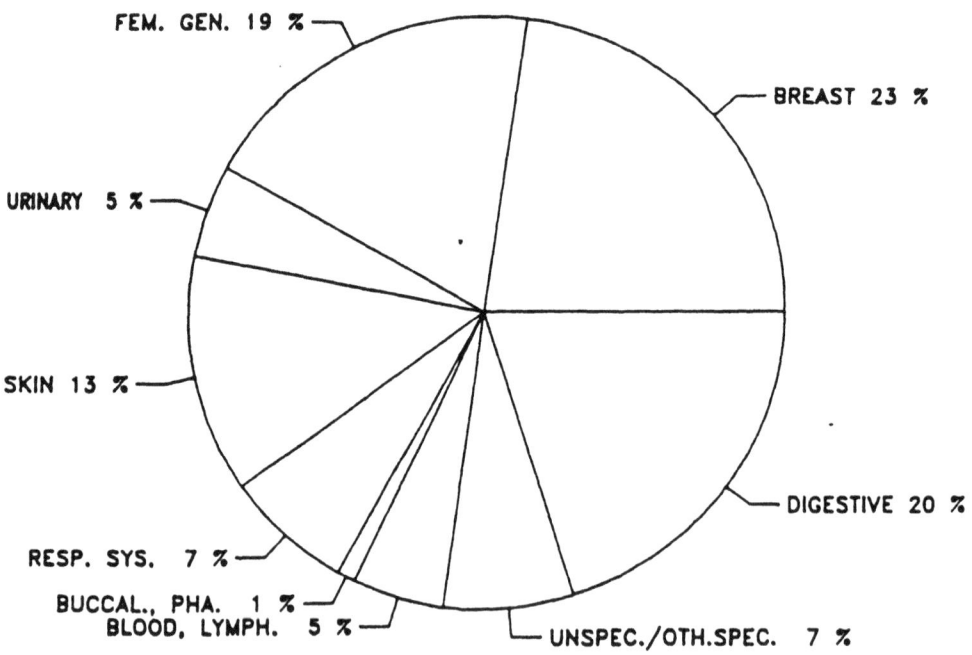

Fig. 1b: Proportional distribution of the age standardized incidence rates (World population) on different organs. Females, 1982.

PRELIMINARY RESULTS FROM A FEASIBILITY STUDY ASSESSING THE COMPARABILITY
OF DIETARY INFORMATION COLLECTED IN DIFFERENT POPULATION SURVEYS
FOR POSSIBLE USE IN A POOLED COHORT STUDY ON THE OCCURRENCE OF CANCER

H. Boeing[1], J. Wahrendorf[1], C. Thiel[2], L. Heinemann[2], W. Kulesza[3], S.L. Rywik[3]

J. Sznajd[4]

[1] German Cancer Research Centre, Im Neuenheimer Feld 280, 6900 Heidelberg 1, FRG

[2] German Institute for Cardiovascular Research, Berlin-Buch, GDR

[3] Institute for Cardiology, Warsaw, Poland

[4] University of Krakow, Krakow, Poland

INTRODUCTION

Various instruments are available for collecting information on people's dietary habits. Food Frequency Questionnaires (FFQ) are considered to be simple, easily applicable instruments of a semi-quantitative nature yielding an averaged measure of the regularity of consumption of certain major foods. Depending on the circumstances, such questionnaires can comprise from 10 or 15 items to more than one hundred.

24-hour recall is another simple method used when the average consumption of a study population is to be characterized. As it only refers to a single day of an individual's dietary pattern, it cannot be used to characterize the dietary habits of individuals.

Recording of the actual food intake is regarded as the most precise method of estimating the nutritional intake of individuals. A recording period of 3, 7 or more days results in a relatively stable picture characterizing individuals. Quantification can be achieved by estimation, the use of household measures, or weighing. The duration of the recording period may depend on the degree of accuracy desired for the information on certain components of the diet.

Diet history interviews are directed at the general pattern of consumption by means of a detailed interview, and they are generally considered to give a relevant picture of dietary habits prevailing over a longer period of time.

Different types of epidemiological studies require different types of dietary investigations. In cross-sectional studies aimed at describing the dietary consumption habits of a population or subgroups thereof, it is common practice to use 24-hr recall or 3- or 7-day records. The semi-quantitative FFQ is employed in large surveys when extensive instruments cannot be used or only specific food items are of interest. The diet history interview represents a logistic compromise which can serve the need of individual-based epidemiological studies such as cohort or case-control studies.

In the project Multinational Monitoring of Trends and Determinants in Cardiovascular Disease (MONICA), coordinated by the WHO, 3 cross-sectional surveys are carried out in the study population at the start, after 5 years and after 10 years to monitor the prevalence of risk factors in the population otherwise monitored carefully for the occurrence of cardiovascular diseases. In addition to the data collected in some of the centres under the MONICA core protocol, dietary habits are also investigated using 24-hr recall, diet history interviews, or 3- or 7-day records. Since the survey populations also represent potential cohorts for individual-based follow-up studies, the quantitative dietary information collected over a very short period of time requires an additional component about the long-term regularity of dietary habits.

MONICA centres which proposed to use their survey populations for individual-based epidemiological studies therefore conducted food frequency interviews in parallel with quantitative recording. Since single national or regional MONICA cohorts may still be too small to yield the appropriate number of events required in, for example, cancer epidemiology, a pooling of such cohorts should be considered. This, however, requires comparable exposure information and has led to a feasibility investigation as to whether different quantitative and semi-quantitative dietary methods used in different MONICA centres can lead to comparable characterization of individuals' dietary habits, with sufficient intra- and intercentre variation.

In this paper we report on the investigations carried out with the dietary information collected in the first MONICA surveys in the German Democratic Republic (GDR) and in Poland. In the GDR all 3500 participants filled in a short FFQ, and a subsample of 800 persons completed 3-day records. In the 2 Polish study areas, urban Warsaw and the rural Tarnobrzeg region, the participants, approximately 2600 in each centre, completed a longer FFQ and gave 24-hr recall. Data from these surveys are presented here with a view to comparing the relative performance of the 2 different instruments used.

MATERIALS AND METHODS

The FFQ used in the first GDR-MONICA survey comprised 12 items (consumption of beef, pork, poultry, green leafy vegetables, red and yellow vegetables, raw vegetables, salads, fruit, cereals, rye bread, beer, wine and spirits) and allowed 6 frequency categories of response (days per week: 7, 5, 3, 1, 1/2, 0). Three-day records were kept on a prepared form on which the consumption of about 25 food categories could be noted, including their portion sizes.

A comparison list had been drawn up to ascertain which items from the 3-day record provide a quantification of each of the FFQ items. If necessary, the appropriate proportions of 3-day items contributing to FFQ items were established.

The FFQ used in both Polish centres comprised 38 items, and the open 24-hr recall interviews used codes for about 500 foods and 300 composite meals. The food content of the latter was known through detailed recipes. Again a comparison list had been drawn up to see which items from the 24-hr recall interview refer to each of the items studied in the FFQ.

Within the subsample of participants in the GDR who filled in both instruments and all participants in the Polish surveys, the following analyses were performed: For all individuals of the same age category (covering 10 years each), of the same sex and reporting the same frequency of consumption of a given food item of the FFQ, the quantitative records (24-hr recall or 3-day records) were reviewed to find out whether on those days the corresponding foods were consumed and if so in what quantity. Therefore, for each food frequency category, age- and sex-specific information about the actual frequency of intake and the daily amount of consumption was available and was compared with the information from the questionnaire. By using the expected number of reporting days, based on the information derived from the FFQ, a ratio can be calculated which estimates on the group level the degree of over- or underestimation in the questionnaire-derived information alone for each frequency category.

RESULTS

In Tables 1 and 2 we give the age- and sex-distribution of the whole study populations in the GDR and Poland and the subsample in the GDR who filled in the 3-day records in addition to a FFQ. For further calculations it was observed that, in most instances, age- and sex-specific influences were negligible, and a combined analysis was adequate to describe the data. Since the analysis is still at the preliminary stage, only examples demonstrating the general strategy can be given. In Table 3 we report the actual proportion of possible reporting days found in the quantitative 3-day records for the study participants filling in both instruments in the GDR, for each frequency category of the FFQ. For example, the second entry of the second line, 0.17, indicates that individuals who state that they eat poultry 5 times a week were found to have consumed this item on 17% of the reporting days. The last line in this table gives the values we expect by taking literally the responses in the food frequency categories. For example, for the food frequency category 5 times/week we expect that on 5 out of 7 recorded days (0.71) this item was consumed.

A ratio of the actually observed and the expected reporting days for a given food item can be calculated, and this provides information about the relative performance of the FFQ. The ratios found in the GDR data are shown in Table 4. For example, the second entry in Table 4, 1.37, indicates that individuals reporting a consumption of meat products 5 times weekly — who would therefore be expected to have a proportion of 5/7 = 0.71 but whose actual proportion of consumption days was found to be 0.98 — have a 1.37-fold (0.98/0.71) higher actual consumption than expected. Thus, values above 1 indicate that the information derived by the FFQ may well be an underestimation of the actual consumption, whereas values under 1 signal an overestimation by the FFQ.

For one item, consumption of fresh fruit, we report in Tables 5 and 6 information about the frequency-specific average daily consumption. Table 5 refers to the GDR, and Table 6 to the rural Polish centre, Tarnobrzeg, supervised by Krakow University. Age-, sex-, and frequency-specific average daily consumption was derived by computing the median of the respective strata specific consumptions. Since these medians were fairly stable over age and sex within one frequency category, the means of these age- and sex-specific median intake values are used for summarizing purposes. In Table 5, line (a), it can be seen that in the GDR these means were found to be constant for all food frequency categories. The second line (b) of Table 5 was taken from

Table 3, giving the proportion of actual consumption days found for individuals reporting the respective food frequency categories. The third line (c) gives the proportion of reporting days one would expect based on the food frequency information only. In the fourth line (d) the long-term average daily consumption is computed using the quantification from line (a) and the frequency from line (b), both derived from the quantitative instrument. In contrast, the fifth line (e) gives a corresponding value if the frequency as reported by the FFQ were used. The last line (f) of this table gives the number of individuals in the total study population found in the respective food frequency categories. Computing for this total study population, the weighed average intake using the respective quantifications in line (d) or (e) yields values of 70 g or 113 g per day. The information found in the statistical yearbook of the GDR for 1985 for average daily fruit consumption was 103 g per day.

The same analysis for the rural Polish centre is reported in Table 6. In this case there was some variation in the average daily consumption associated with individuals reporting different frequencies of consumption on the FFQ. Again, using the questionnaire-reported frequency categories, a broader range of long-term average daily consumption (line (e)) was found as compared to the approach using the actual proportion of reporting days as a measure of frequency (line (d)). With the frequency of study participants found in the FFQ categories (last line (f)) one can compute the average population intake values for the whole population. This results in an estimate of 126 g per day using the observed frequencies and 170 g per day using the reported frequencies.

DISCUSSION

This paper illustrates briefly some results obtained during the analysis of dietary information collected in different survey populations. The linking element of these different surveys was that they used both a food frequency questionnaire and a quantitative reporting method (24-hr recall or 3-day record). However, the list of items used in these instrument was different from country to country.

This situation, in which 2 different instruments were filled in by the study participants, provides the possibility of comparing these instruments with each other. The results outlined in Tables 3 and 4 illustrate the relative performance of the FFQ in comparison with the 3-day record method as used in the GDR. It is apparent that interviewees reporting a very frequent (daily or 5 times a week) consumption of certain food items on the FFQ tend to overestimate the actual consumption by this reporting, whereas interviewees reporting less frequent (once a week or every second week) of certain items may actually underestimate the actual consumption. The frequency category for which the information given by the FFQ and the 3-day records coincide varies from food item to food item. As can be seen in Table 4 for items which are fairly widely consumed in a given population, for example meat, meat products or vegetables, the point of turnover, characterized by a ratio of 1.00, can be located higher up on the frequency scale. On the other hand, for items which appear to be less frequently consumed, such as fruit or whole grain bread, the point where an overestimation turns into an underestimation is much further down on the frequency scale. This aspect is also illustrated for beverages where beer, which is a more common beverage, shows a turnover from over- to underestimation in the higher frequency categories, whereas for wine and spirits this is at the lower end of the scale.

In Tables 5 and 6 we have illustrated the consequences of using either the reported frequency from the FFQ or the actually observed proportion of reporting days from the 3-day record or 24-hr recall as a basis for combining the quantitative information with the frequency information. This is illustrated in this paper using the consumption of fruit, an item comparable between the surveys in the GDR and Poland. As already indicated above, the calculation of age-, sex-, and frequency-specific average daily consumptions led to little age and sex variation in either population, and we consequently averaged over these 2 additional strata. The resulting frequency-specific estimate of fruit consumption, if consumed, was 140 g per day for all frequency categories in the GDR, whereas in the rural Polish population there was some variation between 184 and 248 g per day. Possible explanations for this difference will be discussed below. Using the two different survey methods concerning the frequency of consumption, different ranges of daily intake are derived. With the frequency information reported in the FFQ, the range will be from 1 to 140 g per day, whereas using the actually observed proportion of reporting days, the range will be from 14 to 87 g per day in the GDR. Correspondingly the ranges in the rural Polish study population are from 1 to 248 g or from 52 to 161 g. Using these two different versions of frequency-specific average daily consumption in both populations and weighing it by the respective distribution of the study population (given in the last line (f) of tables 5 and 6) two different estimates of the average daily consumption of the population can be derived in each survey. In both populations the estimate is lower if the actually observed proportions of consumption days were used instead of the food frequency information.

There are several possible reasons for the considerably higher value for fruit consumption found in the rural Polish population compared to the study population in the GDR. The 3-day records used in the GDR were kept on forms for a selected number of items, including fruit, and a pre-categorized quantification was requested, whereas in the Polish survey an open 24-hour recall was carried out giving much more flexibility for reporting various food items. The uniform performance of the 3-day record in the GDR may well be due to this aspect of the instrument by which the dietary intake is measured, and could also have caused a systematic under-reporting of the actual intake. Intake of minor quantities may easily be omitted from reporting when subjects are asked to fill in forms with pre-specified categories of food items referring to particular meals. A difference in fruit consumption between the GDR and rural Poland, on the scale found in this investigation, cannot conceivably reflect the real situation, but must be attributed to a large extent to the two different instruments used.

Although the values of the frequency-specific average daily consumptions in the GDR and Poland, as given by line (d) in Tables 5 and 6, are considerably different, it must be noted that they span roughly similar ranges. In the GDR the range is 87 -14 g/day = 73 g/day, whereas the range in rural Poland is 161 -52 = 109 g/day. One should consider that, in an epidemiological cohort study combining several subcohorts, cancer cases are compared with disease-free controls from the same subcohort and that the difference in their respective quantitative exposure variables is used for the estimation of relative risks. The differences in average daily intake assigned to individuals through their respective response categories on the FFQ is found to be of comparable magnitude between the GDR cohort and the rural Polish cohort. This observation made between two subcohorts for a single food item has to be expanded further. The above points would speak in favour of combining subcohorts to a larger cohort, even when the absolute values of the exposure variables for interest may well be systematically different due to different instruments of reporting, as long as the difference of respective categories is of the same order of magnitude between the subcohorts.

Table 1. Age and sex distribution of whole study population (FFQ) and subsample (additionally a 3-day record) in the GDR-MONICA survey, 1983

Age group	Whole study population		Subsample with 3-day record	
	Male	Female	Male	Female
< 35	463 (27%)	455 (25%)	106 (27%)	104 (23%)
35 – 44	523 (30%)	500 (27%)	104 (27%)	134 (30%)
45 – 54	449 (26%)	488 (27%)	114 (29%)	115 (25%)
> 55	303 (17%)	381 (21%)	68 (17%)	100 (22%)
All ages	1738 (100%)	1824 (100%)	392 (100%)	453 (100%)
Total	3562		845	

Table 2. Age and sex distribution of the two MONICA survey populations in Poland, Warsaw and Tarnobrzeg, 1984 (all participants with FFQ and 24-hr recall)

Age group	Warsaw		Tarnobrzeg	
	Male	Female	Male	Female
34 – 44	379	405	375	470
45 – 54	423	429	429	503
55 – 65	463	472	421	459
All ages	1265	1306	1225	1432
Total	2571		2657	

Table 3. Proportion of actually observed reporting days from 3-day record by food item and frequency category (from FFQ) in study participants of the GDR-MONICA survey, 1983, who filled in both instruments

Food group	Food item	Food frequency category					
		Daily	5 x weekly	3 x weekly	1 x weekly	2 x monthly	< 1 x monthly
Meat and meat products	Meat and meat products	0.98	0.98	0.86	0.94	-	-
	Poultry	0.14	0.17	0.11	0.08	0.05	0.03
Vegetables	All vegetables	0.78	0.73	0.72	0.61	-	0.50
	Raw vegetables	0.39	0.39	0.30	0.32	0.24	0.21
Fruit	Fruit	0.62	0.40	0.26	0.19	0.10	0.13
Cereals	Unprocessed cereals	-	-	-	-	-	-
	Whole grain bread	0.25	0.25	0.22	0.16	0.13	0.07
Beverages	Beer	0.89	0.75	0.51	0.28	0.11	0.07
	Wine	0.44	0.38	0.27	0.14	0.09	0.03
	Spirits	0.43	0.39	0.33	0.26	0.14	0.09
Expected proportion of food intake according to food frequency category		1.00	0.71	0.43	0.14	0.07	0

- : no information (total number < 5)

Table 4. Ratio of actually observed reporting days (from 3-day record) to expected reporting days (from FFQ) by food item and frequency category (from FFQ) in study participants of the GDR-MONICA survye, 1983, who filled in both instruments

Food group	Food item	Food frequency category				
		Daily	5 x weekly	3 x weekly	1 x weekly	2 x monthly
Meat and meat products	Meat and meat products	0.98	1.37	2.00	6.17	-
	Poultry	0.14	0.24	0.26	0.54	0.75
Vegetables	Vegetables	0.78	1.02	1.68	4.18	-
	Raw vegetables	0.39	0.54	0.71	2.26	3.50
Fruit	Fruit	0.62	0.57	0.62	1.29	1.00
Cereals	Unprocessed cereals	-	-	-	-	-
	Whole grain bread	0.25	0.95	0.51	1.16	1.89
Beverages	Beer	0.89	1.04	1.19	2.00	1.42
	Wine	0.44	0.53	0.67	1.00	1.18
	Spirits	0.43	0.55	0.77	1.69	2.04

- : no information (total number < 5)
Values < 1 : overestimation through FFQ
Values > 1 : underestimation through FFQ

Table 5. Consumption of fruit in the GDR-MONICA survey, 1983, by FFQ-categories

	Food frequency categories					
	Daily	5 x weekly	3 x weekly	1 x weekly	2 x monthly	> 1 x monthly
(a) Mean of age- and sex-specific median food intake	140	140	140	140	140	140
(b) Proportion of actually observed reporting days	0.62	0.40	0.26	0.19	0.10	0.13
(c) Proportion of expected reporting days (FFQ)	1.00	0.71	0.42	0.14	0.07	0
(d) Average daily intake (g/day) (based on observed reporting days) (a) x (b)	87	56	36	27	14	18
(e) Average daily intake (g/day) (based on FFQ information only) (a) x (c)	140	99	59	20	10	1
(f) Distribution of study population (number)	2209	556	552	67	30	105

Table 6. Consumption of fruit in the Tarnobrzeg-MONICA survey, 1984, by FFQ-categories

	Food frequency categories					
	Daily	5 x weekly	2-3 x weekly	1 x weekly	1-2 x monthly	1 x monthly
(a) Mean of age- and sex-specific median food intake	248	222	200	206	184	224
(b) Proportion of actually observed reporting days	0.65	0.49	0.40	0.34	0.28	0.32
(c) Proportion of expected reporting days (FFQ)	1.00	0.71	0.36	0.14	0.05	0
(d) Average daily intake (g/day) (based on observed reporting days)	161	109	80	70	52	72
(e) Average daily intake (g/day) (based on FFQ information only) (a) x (c)	248	158	72	29	9	1
(f) Distribution of study population (number)*	1389	394	393	208	68	149

*56 participants were not considered in the calculations (they filled in the frequency category "1 time within 10 days" which was offered in the Polish FFQ but infrequently used).

SECTION II

Dietary Assessment Methods for Epidemiological Studies

METHODOLOGICAL STUDY FOR THE VALIDATION OF TWO SELF-ADMINISTERED DIETARY QUESTIONNAIRES IN FINLAND. RESULTS AND PRACTICAL IMPLICATIONS FOR EPIDEMIOLOGICAL STUDIES

P. Pietinen

National Public Health Institute, 166 Mannerheimintie, 00280 Helsinki, Finland

In order to prepare for collaboration between the US National Cancer Institute and the Finnish National Public Health Institute on studies of nutrition and cancer, a long comprehensive self-administered food use questionnaire containing a picture booklet with photos of portion sizes was developed (Pietinen et al., 1987), as well as a short food frequency questionnaire (Pietinen et al., 1987) targeted at a select group of nutrients (total, saturated and polyunsaturated fat, vitamins A, C and E, dietary fibre and selenium). The studies of validation (against 12 two-day records in 190 men) and reproducibility (three administrations each of dietary history in 121 men and food frequency in 107 men) were conducted in March-October 1984 in Helsinki with males aged between 55 and 69.

The results of the validation study showed that the food use questionnaire is a useful tool moderately suitable for assessing usual intake of the 35 nutrients and 17 food groups examined on all levels of analysis. Spearman correlation coefficients range from 0.41 for vitamin A to 0.83 for alcohol. On average, 51% of subjects in the lowest quintile based on the food records were also in the lowest quintile in the food use questionnaire, and 76% were in the lowest two questionnaire quintiles. The figures for the upper tail of the distribution were similar. As for the reproducibility of the food use questionnaire, the intraclass correlation coefficients range from 0.56 for vitamin A to 0.88 for alcohol, with most between 0.60 and 0.70.

The results of the reproducibility study of food frequency questionnaire showed that for single foods, the average level of exact agreement in reporting the same frequency category at least twice was 53%, with improvement to 87% for agreement within one category. The intraclass correlations varied from 0.52 for vitamin A to 0.85 for polyunsaturated fats. In the validity study, correlations between the intake values based on food records and food frequency ranged from 0.32 for vitamin A to 0.61 for polyunsaturated fats. On average, 40-45% of the subjects in the lowest quintile based on food records were also in the lowest quintile in the food frequency questionnaire, and 70-75% were in the lowest two questionnaire quintiles, respectively.

Comparison was made between the food use and food frequency questionnaires in terms of advantages and disadvantages. Correlations between nutrient intake values based on the food use questionnaire and those based on the food frequency questionnaire were relatively high, indicating that the two methods largely capture the same variation in intake. The partial correlations between food record and food use questionnaire values, controlling for food frequency questionnaire values were significantly different from zero for all nutrients examined. The partial correlations were generally about 0.4, with retinol and selenium being the lowest, 0.27 and 0.31, respectively. The partial correlations between food record and food frequency questionnaire values, controlling for the food use questionnaire, were significantly different from zero only for retinol, saturated fat, polyunsaturated fat and fibre.

In conclusion, the food frequency questionnaire is obviously a useful instrument in intervention trials for monitoring qualitative changes in diet, since its reproducibility is high. On the other hand, the food use questionnaire is better suited to the assessment of an individual's "whole diet".

REFERENCES

Pietinen, P., Hartman, A.M., Haapa, E., Rasanen, L., Haapakoski, J. Palmgren, J., Albanes, D., Virtamo, J. & Huttunen, J.K. (1987) Reproducibility and validity of dietary assessment instruments: I. A self-administered food use questionnaire with a portion size picture booklet. Manuscript (submitted)

Pietinen, P., Hartman, A.M., Haapa, E., Rasanen, L., Haapakoski, J., Palmgren, J., Albanes, D., Virtamo, J. & Huttunen, J.K. (1987) Reproducibility and validity of dietary assessment instruments: II. A qualitative food frequency questionnaire. Manuscript (submitted)

THE PROBLEM OF MEASUREMENT ERROR IN CANCER EPIDEMIOLOGY, WITH PARTICULAR REFERENCE TO COHORT STUDIES OF DIET

J. Kaldor

International Agency for Research on Cancer, 150 cours Albert-Thomas, 69372 Lyon Cedex 08, France

Introduction

Over the past two or three decades, considerable progress has been made in the methodological aspects of cancer epidemiology, particularly with regard to study sample selection, and statistical techniques. We have now reached the point where we have a clear idea of the potential sources of bias and confounding, and various strategies in both design and analysis available to avoid them.

Nevertheless, in certain areas, notably the study of diet and cancer, progress has been limited by the difficulties in measuring the variables which one would wish to study as risk factors. In case-control studies, measurement is further complicated by the likely effect of the disease state, not only on the current level of risk factors but on perception and recall of past levels. On the other hand, cohort studies carried out in real time (as opposed to those done historically or retrospectively) offer the possibility of collecting repeat measures of risk factors in healthy individuals. In this paper, we outline the nature of the measurement problem, and describe some ways in which repeat measurement of risk factors can be used to solve it.

Definition of measurement error

The term "measurement error" has traditionally been used in a rather narrow sense, to mean the purely random variation associated with a particular measuring instrument. Although this concept has a parallel in epidemiological research, measurement error can also be interpreted in a much wider sense. We distinguish three different sources of measurement error.

(1) <u>Error due to one's inability to measure the true risk factor</u>. In fact, most of the variables measured as putative risk factors in cancer epidemiology are surrogates for some underlying variable which either has not yet been identified, or is impossible to measure with available instruments. If the variable being measured is correlated, but not identical, with the true risk variable, the relationship between the two may be thought of as measurement error. An example is provided by dietary fat. There is still no universally accepted hypothesis about what metabolic consequence of fat consumption should be proposed as the putative carcinogenic risk factor, and even if there were, it could not be measured at the level of the target cell. One therefore relies on various surrogate variables, such as, in increasing order of surrogacy, blood lipid measurements, food samples analyzed for fat content, a food diary converted to fat content by standard tables, or a dietary recall questionnaire converted by standard tables.

(2) <u>Error due to within-subject variations in the risk factor</u>. Generally, both true and surrogate risk factors share the property that they vary in time within individuals. A measurement made at one point in time may therefore not be representative of the subject's exposure history. It can, however, be viewed as an inaccurate measurement of exposure. Within-subject variation may

follow a long-term trend, such as a gradual decrease in meat consumption with age; it may be cyclic, as illustrated by the seasonal availability of food items, for example, or it may be rather random, as might occur for dietary items if consumption is determined by short-term decisions and tastes. The relative importance of these three types of variation will differ among individuals, and among cultures. In the case of dietary studies, there will also be substantial differences among nutrients. One would expect that variation in total caloric intake would be dominated by long-term trends, whereas changes in individual components of caloric intake might have a more substantial short-term component.

(3) <u>Error due to measuring instruments</u>. This form of measurement error has received the most attention in the past. It describes the variation arising in the theoretical situation where one could exactly repeat a measurement, without altering the quantity being measured. For example, a food sample could be taken, divided into several portions, and each portion separately analyzed for a particular nutrient. The resulting variation among the portions would be entirely due to the analytic technique, if it were reasonable to assume that the food sample was homogeneous. For instruments which depend on subjective response, it is impossible to obtain true repeats of this kind, since there is an inevitable learning process taking place with each repetition.

Mathematical formulation of measurement error

Suppose that we are studying a <u>variable F</u> as a cause of cancer. A measurement of F can then be defined as any <u>measurable variable M</u> which is not independent of F, but which, conditional on <u>F</u>, is independent of the risk of cancer (Risk of cancer = C). In other words, if one knew the value F for an individual, knowing the value of M would not be of any further use in predicting the individual's cancer risk: all relevant information is contained in F. There is no causal association between M and C, but both M and C are causally dependent on F.

All three types of measurement error from the previous section can be expressed in this way. A surrogate measurement of a true risk factor has no independent effect on cancer risk. If a risk factor varies over time within an individual, F would represent the cumulative exposure over some appropriate interval, and M would be simply the exposure over a more limited period, which would be irrelevant in predicting risk were F itself known. Instrument error fits most naturally into this framework, since by definition it is a purely random component superimposed on the factor being measured, and as such, clearly has nothing to do with the risk of cancer.

While being useful conceptually, this definition of measurement error based on conditional independence alone is too general to be applied directly in mathematical modelling. The two examples which follow are of more specific mathematical formulations of measurement error, and they will be used subsequently to illustrate solutions to the measurement problem.

<u>Continuous risk factor and measurement</u>. Suppose the true risk factor F has a continuous distribution in the study population, and that conditional on F, the measurement M has expected value F, and variance v_M. The measurement is thus, on average, unbiased, although it is also possible to build in measurement bias to the model, and at each value of F in the study population, its variance has a constant value. In order to satisfy the definition of a measurement, M must be independent of the risk of cancer, conditional on F.

<u>Dichotomous risk factor and measurement</u>. Suppose now that F is dichotomous, with prevalence p in the study population, and M is a measurement of F with sensitivity s_1 and specificity s_2. Sensitivity and specificity refer to the probability that M correctly measures F when F is present and absent, respectively. The values of s_1 and s_2 must not be related to disease status, or else the conditional independence of M and C does not hold. This requirement is violated in case-control studies when there is a recall bias, but should be satisfied in cohort studies, where risk factors are measured before the onset of disease.

The effect of measurement error on epidemiological inference

It has been known for many years that when a variable is measured with error, its apparent relationship with other variables is weakened (Bross, 1954). In particular, if a risk factor is subject to measurement error, the apparent strength of its effect in disease risk will always be less than its real effect. Under assumptions of normality on the distribution of a continuous risk factor F and its measurement M, it can be shown that if F is linearly related to the logarithm of disease risk, with slope parameter b, M also has a log-linear relationship to relative risk, but with a smaller slope b'. The extent to which the slope is reduced is expressed by

$$b' = b \cdot c,$$

where $c = v_F / (v_M + v_F)$, and v_F

is the variance of F in the study population. Thus the greater the measurement error v_M in relation to the variance v_F, the greater the reduction in apparent slope (Armstrong and Oakes, 1982; Whittemore and Grosser, 1986).

Similarly, if F is a dichotomous risk factor with associated relative risk r, the relative risk between M and C is always less than r, to an extent which depends on s_1, s_2, and p, the prevalence of F in the study population (Tzonou et al., 1986).

As well as reducing the magnitude of effect parameters and hence the power or probability of detecting relationships in epidemiological studies (Walker and Blettner, 1985), measurement error has a more insidious effect when adjustment for confounding is required. If a confounding variable is measured with substantial error, then adjustment for it in the estimation of another variable's effect will not be possible: most of the confounding will remain even after adjustment (Tzonou et al., 1986, Kaldor and Clayton, 1985).

Solutions to the problem of measurement error

The problem of measurement error could be very simply solved if the error parameters were known. One could then use the measurements in the usual way to estimate effect parameters, such as the slope for a continuous risk factor or the relative risk for a dichotomy, and then correct the estimates according to the appropriate formula relating the true parameter to the biased parameter based on the measurements. For example, if the parameters v_F and v_M were known for a continuous risk factor, b' could be estimated from case-control or cohort study data, and the formula relating b' to b then inverted to give an estimate of b. Greenland and Kleinbaum (1983) propose a similar method for dichotomous risk factors.

In practice, however, the measurement error parameters are rarely known. This leaves two other options. Either they can be estimated and then used as if they were known, in the way described above; or they can be treated as additional unknown parameters in a full statistical model describing not only the relationship between risk factors and disease risk, but also the distribution of the risk factors in the population and the measurement error (Clayton, 1987). The first option has the virtue of simplicity, but the second may give more realistic confidence intervals for the parameters of interest, since it takes account of the variance involved in the estimation of the measurement error parameters.

In any case, both approaches require that the error parameters be estimated. For some risk factors which are subject to measurement error, it may be possible given sufficient resources to make an essentially error-free measurement for a sub-group of study subjects. This measurement could then be used as the "gold standard" against which a more easily obtainable, but inexact measurement could be calibrated, and its precision quantified (Elton and Duffy, 1983). Unfortunately, this situation also tends to be the exception. Either the true risk factor is unknown, or it cannot be measured without substantial error. Nevertheless, it is still possible to estimate the measurement error if repeat measurements of the factor are available for at least a sub-group of individuals. The definition of what constitutes a repeat measurement, like that of a measurement itself, can be rather general: two variables M_1 and M_2 may be thought of as repeat measurements of F if they are not independent of F, but are independent of each other conditional on F. The definition includes the kind of repetition implied by dividing samples for duplicate analysis by the same technique, but also includes pairs of variables which may, on the surface seem rather different. For example, in studying whether an infectious agent was the primary cause of cervical cancer, one could view variables such as number of sexual partners and frequency of intercourse as measurements of infection status, in the absence of a specific means for its determination. Both of these variables would be related to the probability of infection, but conditional on infection status, they may well be independent of each other (Kaldor and Clayton, 1985).

Examples

Correction of a slope estimate for a continuous risk factor. Suppose a measurement M is made on n subjects in whom disease status was ascertained, and that b is the estimated slope relating M to the risk of disease. If the subjects are chosen at random from the population, the total variance of M is $v_T = v_F + v_M$, and it can be estimated by

$$\hat{v}_T = \Sigma (M_i - \overline{M})^2 / (n-1),$$

where M_i is the measurement for the ith subject, and $\overline{M}$ is the average over all n subjects. Suppose also that for k study subjects, a repeat measurement of M was made, producing values M_{1j} and M_{2j}.

These k subjects need not be a subset of the n in whom disease status had been determined. Defining $D_j = M_{1j} - M_{2j}$, v_M can be estimated by

$$\hat{v}_M = \Sigma (D_j - \overline{D})^2 / 2(k-1).$$

We thus have an estimate of v_M and v_F can be estimated by

$$\hat{v}_F = \hat{v}_T - \hat{v}_M$$

The slope estimate $\hat{b}$ can then be corrected using the formula (1) above, to give an estimate for the relationship between disease risk and the true exposure variable F.

Martin et al. (1986) measured serum cholesterol among over 360,000 men, who were then followed up for coronary heart disease (CHD) mortality. The cholesterol level in the population was distributed roughly normally, with mean about 211 mg/dl, and variance 2443, which is an estimate of v_T. A separate study of repeat measures gave an estimate of 324 for the measurement error variance v_M, and subtraction from $\hat{v}_T$ gives $\hat{v}_F$. Substitution into the formula (1) results in a correction factor of 1.15 for the estimated slope relating the "true" cholesterol level to CHD mortality.

Modelling error for a dichotomous risk factor

Suppose measurements of a dichotomous risk factor are made in a study of disease. If it is assumed that the misclassification of the risk-factor is independent of disease status, there are four unknown parameters: the prevalence of the true risk factor F, the sensitivity and specificity of the measurement M, and the relative risk relating F to disease status. If only a single measurement of M is available, the observable data fall into the 4 cells of a 2 x 2 table, and the 4 parameters cannot be estimated since there are at most 3 degrees of freedom, and perhaps two if the design is a case-control study. However, if repeat measurements are available, even for a subset of study subjects, all four parameters can be estimated. Clayton (1985) gives the results from a study of exercise and heart disease in which a relative risk of 2.9 was estimated between a dichotomous measurement of exercise and CHD mortality. When repeat measurements taken on a subsample were used to fit the 4 parameter model, the result was an estimate of 5.2 for the relative risk relating the true value of the dichotomy to the risk of death from CHD.

References

Armstrong, B.G. & Oakes, D. (1982) Effects of approximation in exposure assessments on estimates of exposure-response relationships. Scand. J. Work Environ. Health, 8 (suppl. 1), 20-23

Bross, I. (1954) Misclassification in 2x2 tables. Biometrics, 10, 474-486

Clayton, D.G. (1985) The reliability of measurements: implications for the design and analysis of aetiological studies. Statistics in Medicine, 4

Clayton, D.G. (1987) Models for the analysis of cohort and case-control studies with inaccurately measured exposures, (not published)

Elton, R.A. & Duffy, S.W. (1983) Correcting for the effect of misclassification bias in a case-control study using data from two different questionnaires. Biometrics, 39, 659-664

Greenland, S. & Kleinbaum, D.G. (1983) Correcting for misclassification in two-way tables and matched-pair studies. Int. J. Epidemiol., 12, 93-97

Kaldor, J.M. & Clayton, D.G (1985) Latent class analysis in chronic disease epidemiology. Statistics in Medicine, 4, 327-335

Martin, M.J., Hulley, S.B., Browner, W.S., Kuller, L.H. & Wentworth, D. (1986) Serum cholesterol, blood pressure, and mortality: implications from a cohort of 361 622 men. Lancet, ii, 933-936

Tzonou, A., Kaldor, J.M., Day, N.E. & Trichopoulos, D. (1986) Misclassification in case-control studies with two dichotomous risk factors. <u>Rev Epidemiol Sante Publ</u>, 34, 10-17

Walker, A.M. & Blettner, M. (1985) Comparing imperfect measures of exposure. <u>Amer. J. Epidemiol.</u>, <u>121</u>, 783-790

Whittemore, A.S. & Grosser, S. (1986) <u>Regression methods for data with incomplete covariates</u>. In: Moolgavkar, S.H. & Prentice, R.L. eds. <u>Modern Statistical Methods in Chronic Disease Epidemiology</u>, New York, John Wiley & Sons, pp. 19-35

REPRODUCIBILITY AND VALIDITY OF A SELF-ADMINISTERED DIETARY QUESTIONNAIRE

W.C. Willett

Harvard School of Public Health, Channing Laboratory, 180 Longwood Avenue, Boston, MA 02115, USA

In a prospective study on diet and cancer, which represents a major investment over many years, serious consideration should be given to allocating some of the resources to a validation component. There are several reasons for conducting such a substudy, which involves a detailed assessment of diet on a sample of the study population. First, one can use these data to describe the distribution of dietary intake in terms of the true mean and standard deviation of the exposure in the study population. This is obviously important information. One can obtain a mean and standard deviation from the questionnaire used in the total study population; however, the true variation cannot be separated from the variation due to measurement error. Second, when interpreting findings from the study, it will be important to quantify the misclassification associated with the dietary questionnaire that has been employed. Third, as has been discussed by others at this meeting, one can use this information to correct relative risk estimates and other measures of effect. Fourth, one can use information from the validation study to interpret the extent to which confounding by dietary factors has been controlled in the study.

In designing a validation study, the first consideration is the method to serve as the gold standard. An important characteristic of the standard method is that its error should be, to the extent possible, independent from the error in the questionnaire. An assessment of the reproducibility of a dietary questionnaire will not be sufficient, since much of the error will be correlated if one simply administers the same questionnaire twice to the same subjects. Because of the structured nature of a dietary questionnaire, many errors (due to omission of an important food or misinterpretation of an item) are likely to be repeated on a second administration. Thus a questionnaire can be highly reproducible but extremely invalid. We have come to believe that the diet record is probably the optimal choice for a gold standard; it seems that virtually everyone here has come to the same conclusion. The diet record is probably optimal, even though not perfect, for several reasons. First, it does not rely on memory, which is likely to be a major source of error associated with recall methods or any kind of food frequency questionnaire. Second, the diet record allows a direct measurement of serving sizes, hopefully using actual scales or linear measurements. Third, the method is open-ended and therefore allows a detailed description of foods in as much detail as one can extract. Diet records are not constrained in the same way as standardized questionnaires inevitably are. The point made earlier by Dr Kaldor is very important; the days of diet collection should span a meaningful period. We are a bit vague about what the meaningful period is, but certainly consecutive days are not desirable. For practical reasons, multiple days spaced out over a year are probably a reasonable choice, although one might be more interested, if one thinks the true exposure is operative over multiple years, in days sampled over a multiple-year period. These considerations have been incorporated in the several validation studies that we have conducted.

The first validation study we have completed was conducted within the Nurses Health Study (Willett et al., 1985). The questionnaire being evaluated was one that we used for the total cohort in 1980. It was a very short questionnaire: 61 food items that we carefully selected to provide maximal information on 18 specific nutrients. It required 10-12 minutes, on the average, to fill out and was very inexpensive to process. It was mailed and completed self-administered; we did not have any direct contact with the individual subjects. Thus, it was a very low-cost, very simple dietary questionnaire.

From the participants in the greater Boston area who answered this questionnaire, we selected a sample. Of the women that we asked to participate, 194 (90%) agreed. Every three months over the subsequent year, each woman completed a one-week weighed diet record. At the end of the one-year period, they repeated the same questionnaire that was completed at the beginning of the one-year period. We anticipated that the 28 days of diet recording would dampen within-person variation and thus provide a good estimate of individual intake over a one-year period. The repeat questionnaire provided a measure of reproducibility which is useful, although not sufficient in itself. The repeat questionnaire also allowed us to examine the association with the diet records in both directions, in other words, to compare either questionnaire with the total 28 days. This is important since the sequence of measurements in any validation study is problematic; if we compare the questionnaire with diet records during the subsequent year, the true correlation will be underestimated because the questionnaire relates to diet during the previous year. On the other hand, we were concerned that the act of recording diet during a one-year period might influence response to the questionnaire, perhaps in an artifactually favourable way, to the second questionnaire. It is likely that the true correlation should lie somewhere between. Fortunately, in our data, it does not make a major difference whether the diet records are compared with the questionnaires administered before or afterwards; this is reassuring. The correlations tend to be slightly stronger with the second questionnaire, as expected, but the difference is not great.

A validation study of this type generates an enormous amount of data and it is not possible or appropriate to present much of it here. We have examined the data in several ways. One is by simple cross-classification by quintiles where it is assumed that the quintiles defined by the 28 days of diet recording are the gold standard; this categorization is then compared with quintiles derived from the food frequency questionnaire. For example, in the case of calorie-adjusted cholesterol intake, of the 34 women who were in the lowest quintile by the diet record, 18 were also in the lowest quintile according to our simple questionnaire, and 28 out of the 34 were in the lowest one or two quintiles. Only two women were extremely misclassified. Similarly, at the high end of intake, of the 34 people classified in the highest quintile by the diet record, half were also classified as top quintile by the food frequency questionnaire, and 23 out of the 34 were in the highest two quintiles according to the food frequency questionnaire. The same information is expressed, in a very succinct way, by a correlation coefficient. When one is examining many nutrients, being compact is a considerable virtue. The contingency table just described for calorie-adjusted cholesterol intake corresponds to a correlation coefficient of about 0.60.

We have presented our data both with and without adjustment for caloric intake. The process of adjustment for caloric intake has two influences, in opposite directions, on correlations. One effect is to decrease variability between persons (which lowers correlations), the other effect is to cancel out correlated error (which increases correlations). For macro-nutrients we found that, in this data set, the balance fell on the side of increasing correlation coefficients. However, in general, the effect of such adjustment will depend on which of these effects are dominant. Whatever the effect of adjustment for caloric intake on correlations, it is important to present data in this way since nutrient intakes will be of particular interest in epidemiological analyses after accounting for energy intake (Willett & Stampfer, 1986). After such adjustment, correlations in our validation study tended to run from about 0.5 to 0.7, although vitamin A was somewhat lower.

The questionnaire used in the Nurses Health Study in 1980 (which was the subject of the validation study just described) was constrained in length since our data entry costs were rather large. After conversion to optical scanning we were somewhat less restricted in the length of the questionnaire. Initially, we were also worried about response rate; however, we have subsequently found that people do not hesitate to complete longer forms. They are generally interested in diet and willing to answer more extensive questionnaires than we had originally thought. We therefore expanded our questionnaire to about 120 items. It is more refined in the sense that foods are less grouped together and is somewhat more complete.

We have had several opportunities to evaluate this revised questionnaire. In 1984 we re-contacted the same women who participated in the original validation study (Willett et al., in press). Of these, 150 women completed this more comprehensive food frequency questionnaire. As with the original questionnaire, it was self-administered and completed by mail; no personal contact was involved in filling out the form. We compared this revised questionnaire with the diet records completed four years earlier and found correlations that were quite similar to those for the questionnaire completed at the end of the diet recording period. One would anticipate lower correlations due to the longer interval; our interpretation is that the questionnaire has been improved enough to compensate for about three years of memory loss. We do not know how much the correlations would have decreased if we had used the same questionnaire, so this is only qualitative reassurance that the questionnaire has probably been improved. These data also provide evidence that one can make meaningful measurements of diet of a three- or four-year period in the past using a simple, self-administered form.

We conducted another small validation study at essentially no cost, capitalizing on a very detailed data set collected by the U.S. Department of Agriculture (Willett et al., 1987). Twenty-seven people kept a diet record continually for a year; obviously we are not going to claim that this population is representative of anyone. A year and a half later, Dr Robert Reynolds told us about this group and suggested that we mail our questionnaire to the participants. This population was more heterogeneous. It included both men and women, and their ages ranged from 20 up to 55 years. This illustrated several interesting points. We examined the crude correlations (i.e. unadjusted for caloric intake) and they were, in general, considerably higher than the crude correlations in our previous study population. However, when we adjusted for age and sex, we removed variability that was simply due to age and sex, and the correlations decreased. Since we will always adjust for age and sex in our epidemiological analyses, our validation analysis should also be conditional on age and sex. Similarly, when we adjusted for caloric intake, correlations decreased to approximately the same degree as when adjusted for age and sex. These data demonstrate the importance of presenting data from validation studies adjusted for age and sex (since this is the epidemiologically useful validity) and caloric intake (since the effects of nutrients independent of total energy intake are of central interest in many studies).

In designing a validation study, another basic consideration is the number of days of diet record that are to be collected per subject. In our original validation study we collected 28 days per subject; other validation studies have used 24 or 18 days. This appears to be sufficient to dampen fairly well the within-person variability for most nutrients. However, this amount of data collection requires an enormous amount of work, is very expensive, and demands a high level of cooperation from the participants. One would like to use a smaller number of days per subject if possible. Unfortunately, there is no universal answer as to how many days are needed. This depends on the within-person variability, which varies by nutrient. For a nutrient with very high day-to-day variation, even 28 days is not optimal.

A quite different option is to collect only a few days per subject and then statistically correct the measure of association between the questionnaire and diet record data for the within-person variability. Such methods for correcting correlation coefficients for within-person variation have been available for decades (Beaton et al., 1979; Rosner & Willett, in press).

To illustrate the feasibility of this procedure, we utilized data from our original validation study and sampled only either two days or four days out of the total of 28 days per subject. We then calculated correlation coefficients between the questionnaire and either two, four, or 28 days of diet record. For sucrose, which has a relatively high day-to-day intra-class correlation ($r = 0.40$), the correlation between the questionnaire and diet record increased as the number of days of diet recording increased. However, the increase was not very dramatic because even two or four days were providing a reasonable representation of sucrose intake. When the observed correlations were corrected for within-person variability, the corrected correlations for two or four days were somewhat higher and very similar to using all 28 days of diet recording. Dr Rosner and I have described a method for calculating the standard error of the corrected correlation coefficient. Although the corrected correlation is similar whether a small or large number of days are used per subject, not surprisingly the standard error is larger if a smaller number of days per subject are used.

While the number of days did not make a great different for sucrose intake, the number of days was very important for cholesterol, which has a much lower intra-class correlation, meaning there is a much greater day-to-day variability in cholesterol. If only two days of diet record were used, the correlation between the food frequency questionnaire and the two days of diet record was only 0.19 for cholesterol. After correction, the correlations for either two or four days of diet record were similar to the correlation using all 28 days ($r = 0.51$). Interestingly, 28 days was still causing some attenuation in our correlation with cholesterol intake since it increased from 0.51 to 0.57 after correction for the within-person variability.

The possibility of using only a small number of days of diet recording per subject raises another interesting question: given a fixed number of days of diet record information, what is the optimal number of days per subject? In other words, if one has enough money in a study to measure X number of days of diet recording, what is the best allocation? Should one try to enroll more subjects and obtain few days per subject, or enroll few subjects and many days of diet record per subject? There are several advantages in using a small number of days per subject. The first is that there is less imposition on the subjects, which is likely to mean more cooperation and higher participation rates. This may apply to dietary record data since unusually cooperative subjects are needed to collect 28 days. This issue is even more critical when using something like 24-hr urines, since it is rather difficult to collect 24-hr urines for more than a few days. Others have calculated that 20 or 30 24-hr urines are needed to represent sodium excretion adequately; this is really not feasible in any sort of normal study population. Another advantage of using fewer observations per subject is that this is less likely to impact on behaviour and on reponses to the instrument (e.g. the questionnaire) being tested.

Dr Rosner and I have examined the issue of the allocation of days; whether a large number of days per subject and few subjects, or few subjects and many days per subject is most statistically efficient. This can be addressed by finding the condition that provides the smallest standard error for the corrected correlation coefficient. There is no simple answer since this depends both on the true correlation and on the inter-class correlation. In most applications, true correlations range from 0.5 to 0.7 and inter-class correlations tend to be about 0.3 to 0.7. Under these conditions, the minimal standard error is usually obtained with only two measurements per subject and the maximum number of subjects. Even where the optimal number is larger than two measurements per subject, there is never any large advantage in obtaining greater numbers of measurements per subject when this requires reducing the number of subjects.

This finding has potentially important implications for conducting validation studies. It is nice to collect a large number of measurements per subject as we did. However, if resources are limited, by using the approach described above, one can still mount useful validation studies since they become affordable in almost any circumstance. Statistical efficiency, of course, is not the only consideration and, as long as a subject is enrolled (there are some initial costs in identifying a subject), it may cost little more to obtain a full 7 days of diet recording per subject. Beyond that amount of data, however, the marginal increase in information from additional weeks starts to decrease rather rapidly.

By providing a quantitative measure of exposure misclassification, validation studies can provide the basis for correcting of relative risk estimates. This may ultimately be their most important function. In the context of dietary questionnaires, this does require a validation study, not simply a repeat measure of the questionnaire. This will be apparent by considering that a questionnaire can be highly reproducible but extremely invalid. This could be the case if, for assessment of fat intake, the wrong questions were asked.

Dr Rosner and I are working on the development of methods to estimate misclassification from a validation substudy and then utilize this information to correct the observed relative risks and their confidence limits for the measurement error. Although it is not strictly a linear function, the typical magnitude of correlation coefficients between questionnaires and diet records (r = about 0.60), means that the excess relative risk (RR -1) will be underestimated by a factor of about two. That is, a true relative risk of 2.0 will be observed as being about 1.5. When designing a validation study to correct relative risk estimates, will it be necessary to consider the appropriate number of participants? We have conducted a series of simulations to determine how the size of the validation study ultimately affects the confidence intervals for the corrected point estimate. Again, there is no single correct answer, since it varies from nutrient to nutrient. It appears, however, that the optimal size for a validation study is probably between 100 and 200 people. Beyond 200 people in the validation study, there is only a very minimal effect on the confidence interval under the conditions of variability that we are usually dealing with. This number assumes that a substantial number of days are obtained per subject; a somewhat larger number of subjects will be needed if few days are collected.

Combining data from multiple studies

One last point relates to an issue raised earlier. What about combining data from different studies? In the case of diet studies, this represents a particular challenge because the between-person variation in dietary factors may be different in each population. Furthermore, our measurement methods will have a varying degree of accuracy from one study to another.

This area requires further methodological development. It seems, however, that a rational approach could be based on validation studies conducted for each cohort. In this way, questionnaires could each be standardized against an absolute measure of intake (preferably corrected for total energy intake). In combining results, relative risk estimates could be corrected for measurement error and then be weighted, not only by the usual observed variance, but also by the accuracy of the questionnaires (which would contribute to the variance). In this manner it would be possible to assign objectively small weights to studies with poor measurements of diet and large weights to studies with excellent measurements of diet.

Summary

From validation studies already completed by several groups of investigators, it is already clear that simple structured questionnaires can provide useful, although far from perfect, measurements of diet in epidemiological settings. If possible, validation studies should be incorporated into major cohort studies since they will provide an important basis for interpreting the ultimate associations that are observed. In the future, data from validation studies are likely to be used to correct observed measures of association for measurement error and, possibly, to provide an objective basis for combining data from different populations. In most instances, diet records will be the best comparison method. If it is not possible to collect many days of information for each subject, even as few as two non-consecutive days can be employed.

REFERENCES

Beaton, G.H., Milner, J., Corey, P. et al. (1979) Sources of variance in 24-hour dietary recall data: implication for nutritional study design and interpretation. Am. J. Clin. Nutr., 32, 2456-2459

Rosner, B. & Willett, W.C. (1987) Interval estimates for correlation coefficients corrected for within person variation: implications for study design and hypothesis testing. Am. J. Epidemiol. (in press)

Willett, W.C., Reynolds, R.D., Cottrell-Hoenher, S. et al. (1987) Validation of a semi-quantitative food frequency questionnaire: comparison with a one-year diet record. J. Am. Diet. Assoc., 87, 43-47

Willett, W.C., Sampson, L., Browne, M.L. et al. (1987) The use of a self-administered questionnaire to assess diet four years in the past. Am. J. Epidemiol. (in press)

Willett, W.C., Sampson, L., Stampfer, M.J. et al. (1985) Reproducibility and validity of a semi-quantitative food frequency questionnaire. Am. J. Epidemiol., 122, 51-65

Willett, W.C. & Stampfer, M.J. (1986) Total energy intake: implication for epidemiologic analyses. Am. J. Epidemiol., 124, 17-27

RESULTS OF THE METHODOLOGICAL STUDY
FOR THE DESIGN OF A SIMPLIFIED, SELF-ADMINISTERED QUESTIONNAIRE

R.A. Bausch-Goldbohm[1], P.A. van den Brandt[2], P. van 't Veer[1], F. Sturmans[2] & R.J.J. Hermus[1]

[1] TNO-CIVO Toxicology and Nutrition Institute, P.O. Box 360, 3700 AJ Zeist, The Netherlands

[2] Department of Epidemiology, University of Limburg, Maastricht, The Netherlands

INTRODUCTION

I would like to discuss the development of the food questionnaire that is being used in the cohort study on diet and cancer in the Netherlands. Although we did not have the means, as some of you do, to perform an extensive methodological study prior to the start of the actual study, we considered ourselves lucky to obtain funding for a modest pilot study. We tried to spend this money as efficiently as possible, and designed a two-year scheme with the intention of 1) studying the feasibility and the logistics of the cohort study, and 2) developing a food questionnaire that would be feasible to administer in a large population to measure the habitual consumption of a large number of food groups and dietary constituents.

QUESTIONNAIRE CONSTRUCTION

The approach chosen in the construction of the questionnaire is summarized in Figure 1.

The starting point was a detailed dietary history. The interview was subsequently transformed into a self-administered questionnaire on the basis of experience with the history. After a test for comprehensibility, the questionnaire was reduced in length by excluding a large number of food items. After a second test, the shortened questionnaire was adapted further to yield the one that was actually used in the cohort study. A sample from the first questionnaire is given in the appendix. This paper emphasizes the methods and results of the reduction of the questionnaire.

Dietary history interview

The purposes of the dietary history were: 1) to create a data set containing detailed data on the habitual food intake of the target population; the data would serve as a reference for reduction of the questionnaire; 2) to obtain clues about the comprehensibility of the questions and the reliability of the answers.

The detailed dietary history was taken by interview from 169 men and women who were comparable to the cohort population as far as age and sampling procedure were concerned. The dietary history was designed for these specific purposes, e.g. cross-checks were built in to make sure that the participants reported correct frequencies. Also, portion sizes of important food items were checked by the interviewer through weighing. In order to minimize the effect of seasonal fluctuations, the reference period of choice covered the whole year preceding the interview. The interview took about two hours, while coding took another three hours. The data were used to calculate average daily intake of foods, food groups and a large number of nutrients (see Van den Brandt, elsewhere in this Report). Furthermore, the two interviewers recorded after each interview their experience with respect to the comprehensibility of the questions; they also checked the accuracy of the reported frequencies according to cross-checks. Their experience was used to proceed to the next stage, the construction of an extensive self-administered questionnaire.

General structure of the questionnaire

The extensive self-administered questionnaire was aimed at containing as much information as the dietary history, but in a different form. To understand the general structure of the questionnaire - which was also applied in the dietary history - one should be informed about the main features of the Dutch dietary pattern. The menu in Table 1 demonstrates a fixed pattern, which has been a helpful feature in designing the self-administered questionnaire. The Dutch population, especially in the age range of the target population (55-69 years), usually takes one hot meal a day which is cooked at home. People do not commonly go outside to have such meals. The sandwich meal is eaten outside the house more often, for example at work. In that case, it is usually prepared at home and brought along. This is an uncommon practice in many other countries, as far as my experience goes. The size of a slice of bread, used for breakfast and the sandwich meal is more or less standard. Between meals, snacks and drinks are taken. The snacks may range from nothing at all up to the main source of energy intake during the day (Table 1).

This review may have given the idea that there is not much variation in the Dutch dietary pattern, an undesirable state of affairs for epidemiological studies. There is, however, apart from variation introduced by differing frequencies and portion sizes, variation due to the fact that substitution processes take place. For example, for the sandwich meal people can either take white bread or wholemeal bread; this substitution introduces considerable variation in dietary fibre intake. Similar phenomena apply to sandwich fillings and to components of the hot meal. Furthermore, consumption of snacks contributes to the inter-individual variation; they can vary for example from fruit to French fries.

The regularities in the dietary pattern of the study population, such as the composition of the hot meal (meat, starchy product, vegetables), can be exploited in order to achieve more accurate estimates of consumption frequencies of food groups and specific food items. The consumption frequencies can be asked at several levels, as is illustrated by the following example:

Level 1: Hot meal (frequency)
Level 2: Vegetables in general (frequency, amount)
Level 3: Specific vegetables (frequency, amount)

It should be possible to obtain a reliable estimate of the number of hot meals per week; once you have the frequency of the hot meal, you have under certain conditions the frequency of vegetable consumption, as vegetables are a component of the hot meal. We also ask for the consumption frequency of specific vegetables, but on this level the frequencies range from once or twice a week to once a month or never. If you were to add up the consumption frequencies of specific vegetables, you might obtain a very unrealistic cumulative frequency. Measuring the consumption frequency of food (groups) at different levels helps to keep the data under control - especially if they are not checked by interviewers. Questions 12 and 13 (appendix) show how this principle was applied to the questionnaire.

Reduction of the questionnaire

The most important requirement of a good questionnaire in etiological research is that it is capable of classifying the subjects in the right order with respect to the determinants of interest, i.e. intake of food (groups) and dietary constituents. Correct estimation of the magnitude of the determinant is of secondary importance. This implies that, if there are no differences in the intake of a particular food (group) in the population, strictly speaking we do not have to know its level of intake. In other words, the population does not contain any information as far as the intake of that particular food (group) is concerned. Thus, only those food items have to be included in the questionnaire that contribute to the variance of the dietary constituent (e.g. nutrient) of interest. The contribution of an item is determined by inter-individual differences in its consumption frequency, the portion size or both. Although we used the contribution to the variance as guideline for the selection of items, the reduced questionnaire contains more questions than strictly necessary. These questions are important in order to maintain the logical structure of the questionnaire and for more general use of, as well as inference from, the data. Also, a particular food item might be interesting as such (e.g. fish). On the other hand, several items that should have been selected according to their contribution to the variance were left out, because it was considered impossible to obtain a reliable answer about their consumption (e.g. sauces).

Linear regression analysis was used to calculate the contribution of the food items to the variance of a set of 16 nutrients, including energy. Contrary to the strategy of, for example Walter Willett (Willett, pp. 71-78 of this Report), we did not use stepwise regression analysis to assess the contribution of each item added. The reason was that our data set - originating from the detailed dietary history - contained too few subjects (169) and too many items (about 1000, taking into account the consumption of the same item on different occasions). In order to avoid meaningless predictors from entering the regression equation, we weighted the items according to their nutrient content, i.e. we used the nutrient contribution of a given set of items as a predictor, rather than the amount of food. Thus, for each nutrient the following equation was used:

$$Y = b(\sum_s X_i C_i) + A + \text{error},$$

in which Y denotes the <u>total</u> individual intake of the nutrient as calculated by all - approximately 1000 - items of the detailed dietary history, X_i denotes the individual intake of a <u>selected</u> item i, and C_i denotes the nutrient concentration of item i. The sum of the nutrient contributions of the selected set of items ($\sum X_i C_i$) was entered in the equation. Thus, a selected set of items is characterized by one regression coefficient (b) and intercept (a) and one R squared.

Results of the reduction cycles

The approach described does not help in starting off the selection process. Entering all possible selections of items in the equation consecutively was found too cumbersome and unpractical. Instead, as a first screening, we divided all food items into 27 food groups and calculated for each food group separately the variance contributed to each of the 16 nutrients. Table 2 gives an example of the results for total fat. You may see, for example, that potatoes do not contribute to the variance in total fat consumption, while milk and milk products do. I would like to draw your attention to meat-and-poultry on the one hand and (processed) meat on the other hand. While the former has a relatively high mean intake but a low coefficient of variation, the situation for the latter is the reverse. The reason for this is that the majority of the population eat meat with their hot meal and the portion sizes do not differ very much, there is not much variation in the intake of that food group. Processed meat, on the other hand, is eaten with sandwiches; some people never eat their sandwiches with ham, for example, while others may eat six slices of bread and ham. As a result, (processed) meat has a much larger R squared than meat-and-poultry, although the absolute intake and the absolute nutrient contribution are lower (Table 2).

For the first selection, all items were included that belonged to a food group that contributed 15% or more (R squared >= 0.15) to one or more of the 16 nutrients. The items belonging to other food groups were either excluded or included after they had been aggregated into a group, i.e. only one or two questions concerning the aggregated food group (e.g. cookies) were inserted. The latter procedure was followed in order to reduce the questionnaire without losing all information on the intake of the food group. To calculate the $\sum_S X_i C_i$ for a particular selected set, an adapted food table had to be made, not only containing specific food items, but also aggregated food items. The composition of each aggregated food item i (C_i) was derived from the component food items as the average composition weighted according to their contribution to the consumption of the subjects in the data set. Table 3 (Cycle 1) presents the R squared for the 16 nutrients for the first selection.

Analysis of residuals revealed 15 subjects having residuals larger than the arbitrarily defined criterion of one population standard deviation for one or more of the 16 nutrients. The food items responsible for the large residuals were subsequently included in the list. Furthermore, some individual portion sizes were replaced by standard sizes (population mean). While the first selection contained an individual portion size for each food item included, the second set reflected the fact that for a number of food items it was unpractical to ask for individual portion sizes. The results corresponding with the second selection are presented in Table 3 - cycle 2. For the following selections, more items were excluded or aggregated, while a few items were added. Also, the usefulness of asking for portion sizes was evaluated. Cycle 4 in Table 3 demonstrates the situation that all individual portion sizes are replaced by standard (i.e. mean) sizes, a clearly unacceptable situation. Cycle 7 reflects the final set of food items, which is much smaller than the first one. It corresponds with the questionnaire used in the last test. The test resulted in minor improvements to the questionnaire, which then became final (Table 3).

Comparing cycle 7 to cycle 1 clearly demonstrates that a substantial reduction in the number of food items (from approximately 1000 to 150) and consequently of the number of questions, does not necessarily imply a substantial loss of information. Although the values of R squared, ranging from 86 to 100%, may seem quite high, I would like to point out that this should be so, because the regression analysis was carried out within one data set. In other words, the errors of $Y (= \sum_{total} X_i C_i)$ and $\sum_S X_i C_i$ are not independent. Comparing the data from the questionnaire as it is actually completed with the dietary history data set will of course produce lower values. This comparison has been done, but the results are not yet available.

Actual experience and validation

Some preliminary remarks are justified on the experience with respect to the actual use of the questionnaire in the cohort study. The questionnaire is quite long (median completion time of the test questionnaire including the non-dietary questions was 60 minutes) and not everybody considers it easy to complete. This will have had some effect on the response rate. However, for the cohort study at hand, we considered it more important to have reasonably detailed information on dietary habits from a smaller cohort than to recruit a larger cohort. It is estimated from a sample of the returned questionnaires that 7% cannot be processed because too many answers are missing.

The actual value of the questionnaire as it is being used in the cohort study will be assessed in two validation studies. The first contains a comparison with a dietary history (interview) in the cohort subjects participating in a case-control study on breast cancer (Van 't Veer et al., 1985), while in the second validation study a sample of the cohort members will be asked to record their intake during a number of days throughout the year.

REFERENCES

van 't Veer, P., van Faassen, A., Egger, R.J., Ockhuizen, T., Hermus, R.J.J. & Sturmans, F. (1985) Dietary selenium status, fat consumption and body composition: a case-control study on the etiology of pre- and postmenopausal breast cancer. In: Joossens, J.V., Hill, M.J. and Geboers, J., eds, Diet and Human Carcinogenesis, Amsterdam, Elsevier, pp. 207-212

Table 1. General Dutch Food Pattern

Usually each day:
- breakfast
- one hot meal (lunch or dinner)
- one sandwich meal
- snacks, drinks

BREAKFAST

- tea, coffee or milk (product)
- sandwiches, crackers, rusks, etc.
  filling: cheese, (processed) meats, peanut butter,
    jam, other sweet products
[- oatmeal or wheatmeal porridge][a]
[- cereal]
[- fruit juice]

HOT MEAL

[- soup]
- meat, poultry or fish
- boiled vegetable and/or raw vegetable
- starchy product: potatoes, rice or pasta
- dessert: milk pudding, yogurt or fruit

SANDWICH MEAL

[- soup]
- coffee or milk (product)
- sandwiches
  filling: cheese, (processed) meats, peanut butter,
    jam, other sweet products, raw vegetables
[- fruit]

---

[a] Components between brackets [ ] are taken irregularly or only by part of the population

Table 2. Average daily intake (weight), contribution to fat intake and contribution to the variance of fat intake (R^2) and of 27 food groups

Food group	Intake (g/day)		Fat intake (g/day)		R^2 [b] (*100)
	Mean	CV[a]	Mean	CV[a]	
Potatoes	140	70	1.1	378	6.0
Vegetables	250	41	0.2	99	0.0
Pulses	8	274	0.1	207	0.1
Fruit	205	74	0.0	0	0.0
Cereals	34	120	0.5	208	1.8
Bread	143	47	3.7	126	0.6
Milk and milk products	328	77	8.9	88	25.0
Cheese	40	75	12.0	77	16.5
Eggs	19	69	1.9	70	5.3
Meat and poultry	78	57	11.6	65	13.1
Fish	13	110	1.0	140	6.2
Visible fats, sauces	49	50	37.0	51	62.0
Soups	103	94	2.5	102	8.5
Dishes	10	152	1.0	159	3.6
Cakes, cookies	41	76	5.7	87	9.6
Sugar, candy	31	112	1.4	263	3.6
Snacks	10	191	3.9	172	7.3
Sandwich filling - salt	2	263	1.1	284	6.6
Sandwich filling - sweet	11	124	0.3	258	2.3
Processed meat	21	116	5.1	135	31.9
Shellfish	1	396	0.0	456	0.1
Non-alcoholic drinks	968	40	0.0	0	0.0
Alcoholic drinks	142	190	0.0	530	1.5
Spices	0	530	0.0	0	0
Soy products	1	530	0.1	463	0.9
Seeds	0	836	0.1	817	0.7
Other	2	372	0.1	425	0.6

[a] Coefficient of variation [(SD/MEAN) * 100]
[b] R^2, resulting from simple linear regression analysis of total fat intake on each food group

Table 3. Results of reduction cycles $(R^2 * 100)^a$

Nutrient	Cycle			
	1	2	4	7
Energy	96	98	47	95
Vegetable protein	79	88	55	86
Animal protein	95	96	50	96
Saturated fat	95	96	56	94
Monounsaturated fat	96	97	52	94
Polyunsaturated fat	89	91	51	90
Cholesterol	96	97	63	96
Mono/disaccharides	95	95	55	92
Polysaccharides	87	95	43	93
Alcohol	99	100	68	100
Calcium	97	98	49	98
Vitamin C	97	96	63	95
Beta-carotene	96	97	63	95
Retinol	93	93	57	91
Cereal fibre	90	92	60	91
Vegetable fibre	79	86	46	86

[a] For explanation, see text

Figure 1.

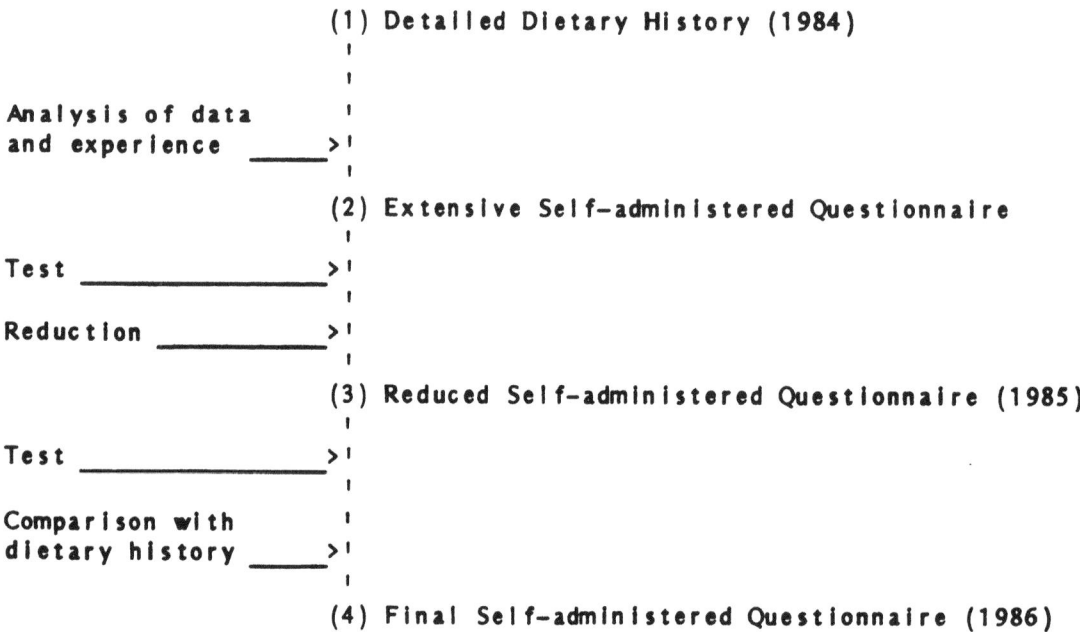

APPENDIX

A sample from the translated questionnaire that is used in the Netherlands Cohort Study on Diet and Cancer

12. How many times per week do you use a hot meal? |_|_| times per week
    Do you prepare the hot meals yourself? O no, seldom or never   O yes |_|_| times per week
    How often did you have these products
    for your hot meal during the past year?

	never or less than 1x per month	1x per mo.	2-3x per mo.	1x per week	2-3x per week	4-5x per week	6-7x per week	how much did you eat?	
* bread instead of a hot meal	O	O	O	O	O	O	O	|_|_|	slices
* Chinese or Indonesian food	O	O	O	O	O	O	O	|_|_|	servingspoons
* Italian food (e.g. pasta, pizza)	O	O	O	O	O	O	O	|_|_|	servingspoons
* soup as main course	O	O	O	O	O	O	O	|_|_|	servingspoons
* fish	O	O	O	O	O	O	O		
* egg instead of meat	O	O	O	O	O	O	O		
* cheese instead of meat	O	O	O	O	O	O	O		
* meat or chicken	O	O	O	O	O	O	O		
* pulses (e.g. white or kidney beans, lentils, marrowfats)	O	O	O	O	O	O	O	|_|_|	servingspoons
* soybean products (e.g. tofu, tempeh)	O	O	O	O	O	O	O	|_|_|	tablespoons
* white rice (not in Chinese food)	O	O	O	O	O	O	O	|_|_|	servingspoons
* brown rice	O	O	O	O	O	O	O	|_|_|	servingspoons
* millet, buckwheat, wheat, barley, oats and other cereals	O	O	O	O	O	O	O	|_|_|	servingspoons
* french fried potatoes	O	O	O	O	O	O	O		
* mayonnaise	O	O	O	O	O	O	O	|_|_|	tablespoons
* potatoes (boiled, fried, mashed or in a mixed dish)	O	O	O	O	O	O	O	pieces the size |_|_| of an egg	
* raw vegetables and boiled vegetables: in winter	O	O	O	O	O	O	O		
in summer	O	O	O	O	O	O	O		
* only raw vegetables without boiled vegetables: in winter	O	O	O	O	O	O	O		
in summer	O	O	O	O	O	O	O		
* only boiled vegetables: in winter	O	O	O	O	O	O	O		
in summer	O	O	O	O	O	O	O		

13. **How often have you used the following vegetables in summer and how often in winter?** Please indicate both frequencies on the same line. If for example you only eat sauerkraut in winter, mark 'never or less than once per month' in summer, and for example 1 time per week in winter. Don't forget to count the vegetables in mixed dishes!

How often did you eat this:	never or less than 1x per month	1x per mo.	2-3x per mo.	1x per week	2x per week	3-7x per week	never or less than 1x per month	1x per mo.	2-3x per mo.	1x per week	2x per week	3-7x per week
	in summer						in winter					
BOILED VEGETABLES												
* brussels sprouts	o	o	o	o	o	o	o	o	o	o	o	o
* leek	o	o	o	o	o	o	o	o	o	o	o	o
* sauerkraut	o	o	o	o	o	o	o	o	o	o	o	o
* cauliflower	o	o	o	o	o	o	o	o	o	o	o	o
* cabbage	o	o	o	o	o	o	o	o	o	o	o	o
* spinach	o	o	o	o	o	o	o	o	o	o	o	o
* endive	o	o	o	o	o	o	o	o	o	o	o	o
* red beets	o	o	o	o	o	o	o	o	o	o	o	o
* carrots	o	o	o	o	o	o	o	o	o	o	o	o
* sliced beans, string beans,	o	o	o	o	o	o	o	o	o	o	o	o
* broad beans	o	o	o	o	o	o	o	o	o	o	o	o
* kale (curly)	o	o	o	o	o	o	o	o	o	o	o	o
RAW AND SWEET VEGETABLES												
* raw endive	o	o	o	o	o	o	o	o	o	o	o	o
* lettuce	o	o	o	o	o	o	o	o	o	o	o	o
* carrot salad	o	o	o	o	o	o	o	o	o	o	o	o
* rhubarb	o	o	o	o	o	o	o	o	o	o	o	o
* apple sauce	o	o	o	o	o	o	o	o	o	o	o	o

14. **How much of the following vegetables did you usually eat?** If you never eat a certain vegetable, fill in 0.

* boiled endive |_|_| grams per person per meal (this is about |_|_| servingspoons
* beans |_|_| grams per person per meal (this is about |_|_| servingspoons
* carrot salad |_|_| servingspoons per meal
* onions |_|_| pieces per week per person
* tomatoes |_|_| pieces per week in summer and |_|_| pieces per week in winter
* mushrooms |_|_| boxes (250 grams) per month per person
* sweet peppers |_|_| pieces per month in summer and |_|_| pieces per month in winter

COMPARISON OF DIETARY HABITS ESTIMATED EITHER BY FOOD FREQUENCY OR FOOD FREQUENCY COMBINED WITH PORTION SIZE

P. Crosignani & C. Mazzoleni

Epidemiology Unit, National Cancer Institute, Via Venezian 1, 20133 Milan, Italy

INTRODUCTION

The dietary history approach is probably the best way to determine an individual's usual food intake (Block, 1982). Various methods have been proposed for selecting food items to be included in a questionnaire so that a reliable quantification of a predefined set of nutrients can be obtained (Willett et al., 1985; Block et al., 1986).

In large prospective studies, a reasonably short self-administered questionnaire is the only feasible solution: in this case care should be taken to collect information in the simplest way and to reach an adequate level of quantification of each food item without superfluous questions.

This paper deals with the problem of finding the questions that should be asked in order to determine the consumption of a single food item using a semiquantitative set of questions, i.e. the frequency of usual intake is recorded directly, whereas for the usual portion size the subject should compare what he/she usually eats with a predefined set of portion sizes.

None of the following considerations are applicable in cases where the quantity can easily be measured as a number of items, e.g. fruit.

MATERIALS AND METHODS

A sample of 118 dietary history interviews (Cubeau & Pequignot, 1980) recorded by trained dieticians from a set of 498 female population controls (Riboli et al., 1987) has been considered. With the interview used, the individual's true intake I of i-th food item is given by:

$$I = \Sigma_j F_{ij} * Q_{ij}$$

where F_{ij} is the j-th frequency of intake of that food and Q_{ij} is the related quantity, considering that one subject can eat different quantities of the same food with different frequencies.

We studied how the true ranking of individuals, the main requisite for analytical studies, is modified by using as a surrogate of the true information the frequency alone, or the frequency plus a multiple-level indication of the quantity, a response that simulates the answer that can be obtained from a semiquantitative food frequency questionnaire.

A detailed description of the misclassification due to the use of surrogate information, is given by the N by N matrix M_{ij}, obtained by subject allocation in an adequate number of N percentiles (e.g. ten deciles) according to both types of information. M_{ij} represents the number of subjects in the i-th category according to the true information, classified in the j-th category using the surrogate information. An overall indicator of the agreement between the two types of information is given by the correlation coefficient (Walker & Blettner, 1985) or by other correlation measures (Willett et al., 1985).

An intermediate level of description between a large matrix and a unique indicator can be obtained by considering the percentage of correctly classified subjects above and below a given percentile of the true variable-defined distribution, according to the surrogate variable distribution. Let ke be a value between 0 and 100, a subject is correctly classified if his/her value is higher (or lower) than the k percentile (k-tile) both in the true and in the surrogate-variable distribution. Let p1(k) be the percentage of the subjects correctly classified below the k-tile and p2(k) the percentage for those classified above the k-tile.

Table 1 and Figure 1 represent p1 and p2 as a function of the parameter k for meat as a food item, using frequency alone as surrogate variable. The misclassification of the subjects appears to be stronger in the highest percentiles.

The main influence of such a non-homogeneous misclassification on the relative risk, besides the bias towards the null (Walker & Bletter, 1985), is the effect on weak dose-response relationships. Table 2 shows how two sets of hypothetical data, with dose-response relationships, among quintiles with different strength, are modified by using the misclassification matrix; the quintiles are determined according to the control distribution.

If the analysis is done by quartile, the influence of this phenomenon appears to be of little importance, as shown in Table 3.

In an attempt to provide a formal framework, and to evaluate whether this lack of homogeneity was inherent to our data or representative of a more general problem, we used a simulation model, supposing that an individual's true intake I of food item i is given by:

$$I = F_i \, v \, Q_i$$

and, considering F_i as surrogate variable, we studied the indicators p1 and p2, as a function of the variability of F_i and Q_i and the correlation between F_i and Q_i. One would expect that, if the variability of Q_i in relation to F_i is high or if Q_i is negatively associated with F_i, the classification one can obtain using F_i instead of the true product will be worse. This simulation model used uniformly distributed random numbers as F_i and Q_i; as an indicator of variability, we used the dimensionless coefficient of variation CV (the ratio between the standard deviation and the mean). Table 4 and Fig. 2 represent p1 and p2 where there is no correlation between F_i and Q_i, with various CVs for the variable Q_i.

These results are in agreement with those obtained in the real situation (meat) and suggest that in cases where the quantity variation is comparable with that of the frequency, the use of frequency alone with no estimate of the quantity can introduce a serious misclassification in the highest percentiles and mask possible trends of the relative risk.

Table 5 and Fig. 3 simulate the situation one may obtain if there exists a correlation between quantity and frequency, when these have the same variability. In the case of a positive correlation, the misclassification is less evident and confined to the higher percentiles whereas, if there is a negative correlation, an important misclassification appears to affect all categories, as shown also by the fall of the indicator p1.

Although a better statistical approach is required in order to provide a more formal framework to these preliminary results, these results seem to have some practical implications.

First of all, one should collect information on the quantity if, and only if, the variation of the quantity itself is comparable to or higher than the variability of frequency or if it appears to be negatively correlated with the frequency. Thus, a pilot study or analysis of previous material collected in the same or in a comparable population is highly fruitful for establishing how many and which questions should be asked for each food item.

The measure of quantity, especially in a self-administered questionnaire is difficult to obtain in conventional units (e.g. grams or fluid ounces). On the other hand, the information on the quantity can easily be obtained by asking the subject to specify whether the amount he/she usually consumes is higher, equal to or lower than a set of predefined amounts. The number of categories one can obtain with L levels of comparison (usually using photographs or shapes) is L v 2 + 1 (see Fig. 4). This semiquantitative way of collecting information on quantity allows the reduction of the residual variability of the quantity at a desired fraction of the variability of the frequency.

Thus, given the number of classes envisaged for the data analysis, one can decide if any information on the quantity should be requested, and how many classes of it should be used, in order to obtain an acceptable classification.

A second implication is that, in view of the possibility of misclassification, it is advisable to use a limited number of classes in the data analysis, especially of a dose-response relationship is of interest.

REFERENCES

Block, G. (1982) A review of dietary assessment methods. *Am. J. Epidemiol.*, 115, 492-505

Block, G., Harman, A.M., Dresser, C.M., Carrol, M.D., Gannon, J. & Gardner, L. (1986) A data-based approach to diet questionnaire design and testing. *Am. J. Epidemiol.*, 124, 453-469

Cubeau, J. & Pequignot G. (1980) La technique du questionnaire alimentaire quantitatif utilise par la Section Nutrition de l'INSERM. *Rev. Epidemiol. Sante Publ.*, 28, 367-372

Riboli, E., Pequignot, G., Repetto, F., Axerio, M., Raymond, L., Boffetta, P., Zubiri, A., Del Moral, A., Esteve, J. & Tuyns, A.J. (1987) A comparative study of smoking, drinking and dietary habits in population samples in France, Italy, Spain and Switzerland. I. Study design and dietary habits. *Rev. Epidemiol. Sante Publ.* (submitted for publication)

Walker, A.M. & Blettner, M. (1985) Comparing imperfect measures of exposure. *Am. J. Epidemiol.*, 121, 783-790

Willett, W.C., Sampson, L., Stampfer, M.J., Rosner, B., Bain, C., Witschi, J., Hennekens, C.H. & Speizer, F.E. (1985) Reproducibility and validity of a semiquantitative food frequency questionnaire. *Am. J. Epidemiol.*, 122, 51-65

Table 1. Meat intake estimated by frequency alone

	Percentiles								
	10	20	30	40	50	60	70	80	90
P1 =	.82	.91	.74	.85	.95	.90	.92	.94	.95
P2 =	.96	.96	.95	.88	.92	.81	.78	.67	.45

Coefficients of variation:
    Quantity 2.89
    Frequency 1.79

Table 2. Modification of dose-response relationships by the misclassification matrix (quintiles)

Example A	Quintile	1	2	3	4	5
	RR	1[a]	1.2	1.4	1.6	1.8
	Misclassification matrix					
		True information-defined quintiles				
	Surrogate information defined quintiles	21	2	0	0	0
		3	14	7	0	0
		0	8	9	7	0
		0	0	8	10	6
		0	0	0	7	16
	(absolute numbers of subjects)					
	RR obtained	1[a]	1.76	1.37	1.56	1.71
Example B	Quintile	1	2	3	4	5
	True RR	1[a]	2.0	3.0	4.0	5.0
	RR obtained	1[a]	2.93	2.72	3.60	4.32

[a] Reference category

Table 3. Modification of dose-response relationships by the misclassification matrix (quartiles)

Example A	Quartile	1	2	3	4
	RR	1[a]	1.2	1.4	1.6
	Misclassification matrix				
		\multicolumn{4}{l}{True information-defined quartiles}			
	Surrogate information defined quartiles	24	5	0	0
		4	22	3	0
		1	3	21	5
		0	0	6	24
	(absolute numbers of the subjects)				
	RR obtained	1[a]	1.28	1.35	1.51
Example B	Quartile	1	2	3	4
	True RR	1[a]	2.0	3.0	4.0
	Obtained RR	1[a]	1.87	2.56	3.23

[a] Reference category

Table 4. Percentage of subjects correctly classified above (p1) or below (p2) a given decile according to different combinations of coefficient of variation, of "quantity" and "frequency" of food consumption. No correlation between "quantity" and "frequency" is assumed.

	Example A	Example B	Example C
CV of the quantity	2.0	1.0	0.5
CV of the frequency	2.0	2.0	2.0
Correlation coefficient	0.0	0.0	0.0

Percentiles

		10	20	30	40	50	60	70	80	90
Example A	p1 =	.87	.87	.87	.87	.87	.87	.88	.90	.94
	p2 =	.99	.97	.94	.91	.87	.80	.71	.61	.46
Example B	p1 =	.93	.93	.93	.93	.93	.93	.92	.93	.95
	p2 =	.99	.98	.97	.95	.93	.89	.82	.71	.54
Example C	p1 =	.96	.96	.96	.96	.96	.96	.96	.95	.96
	p2 =	.99	.99	.98	.97	.96	.94	.91	.82	.66

Table 5. Percentage of subjects correctly classified above
(p1) or below (p2) a given decile according to
different combinations of coefficient of variation,
of "quantity" and "frequency" of food consumption.
Three hypotetical correlation coefficients are
assumed between "quantity" and "frequency".

	Example D	Example E	Example F
CV of the quantity	2.0	2.0	2.0
CV of the frequency	2.0	2.0	2.0
Correlation coefficient	0.4	0.8	-0.5

		Percentiles								
		10	20	30	40	50	60	70	80	90
Example D	p1 =	.88	.89	.90	.90	.91	.92	.92	.92	.95
	p2 =	.99	.97	.96	.94	.91	.87	.81	.70	.54
Example E	p1 =	.88	.90	.92	.92	.92	.92	.93	.94	.95
	p2 =	.99	.98	.97	.96	.95	.91	.90	.81	.68
Example F	p1 =	.74	.69	.67	.68	.71	.75	.80	.86	.93
	p2 =	.97	.92	.86	.79	.71	.62	.54	.44	.34

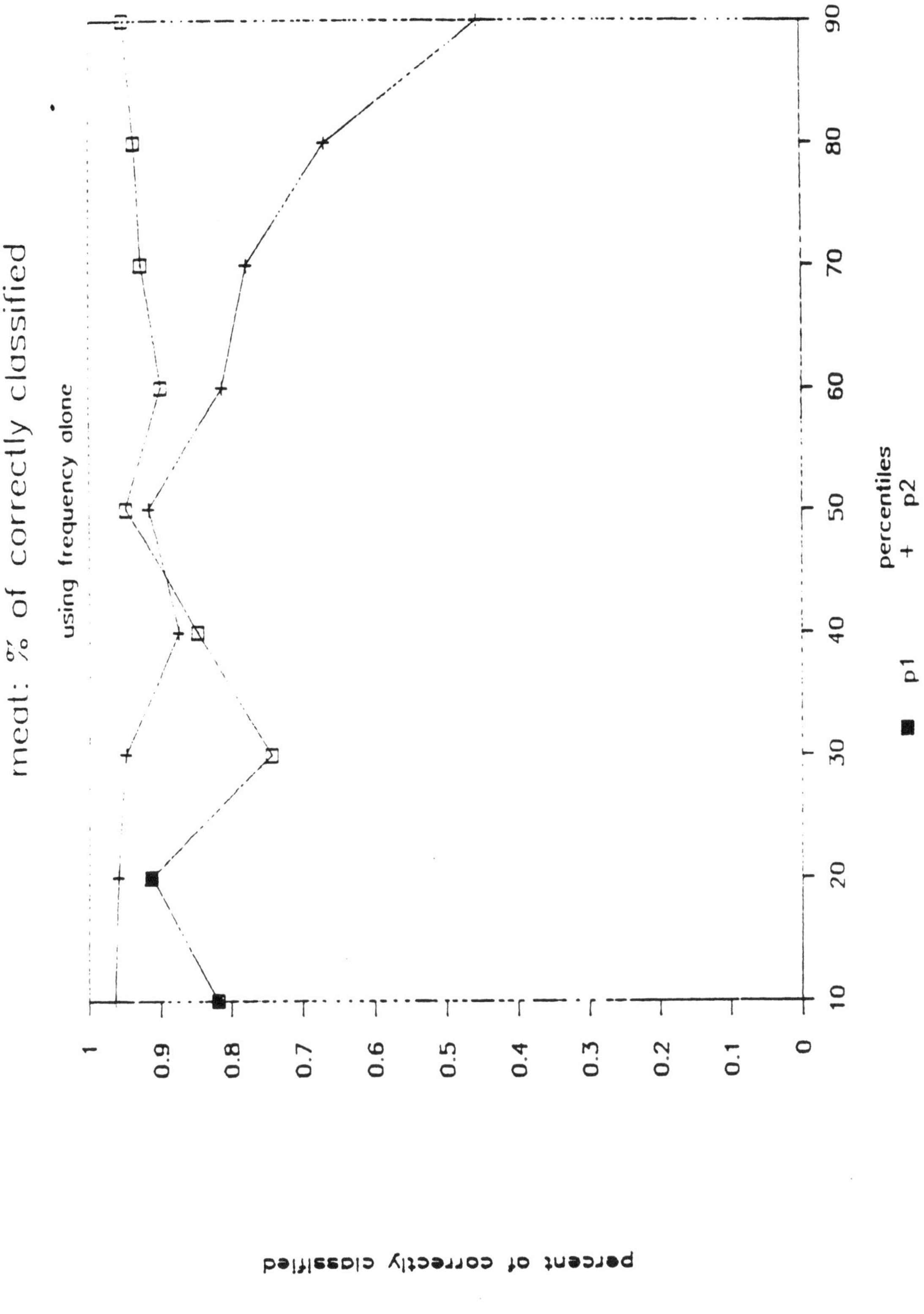
meat: % of correctly classified
using frequency alone
percent of correctly classified
1
0.9
0.8
0.7
0.6
0.5
0.4
0.3
0.2
0.1
0
10
20
30
40
50
60
70
80
90
percentiles
■ p1
+ p2

Figure 1

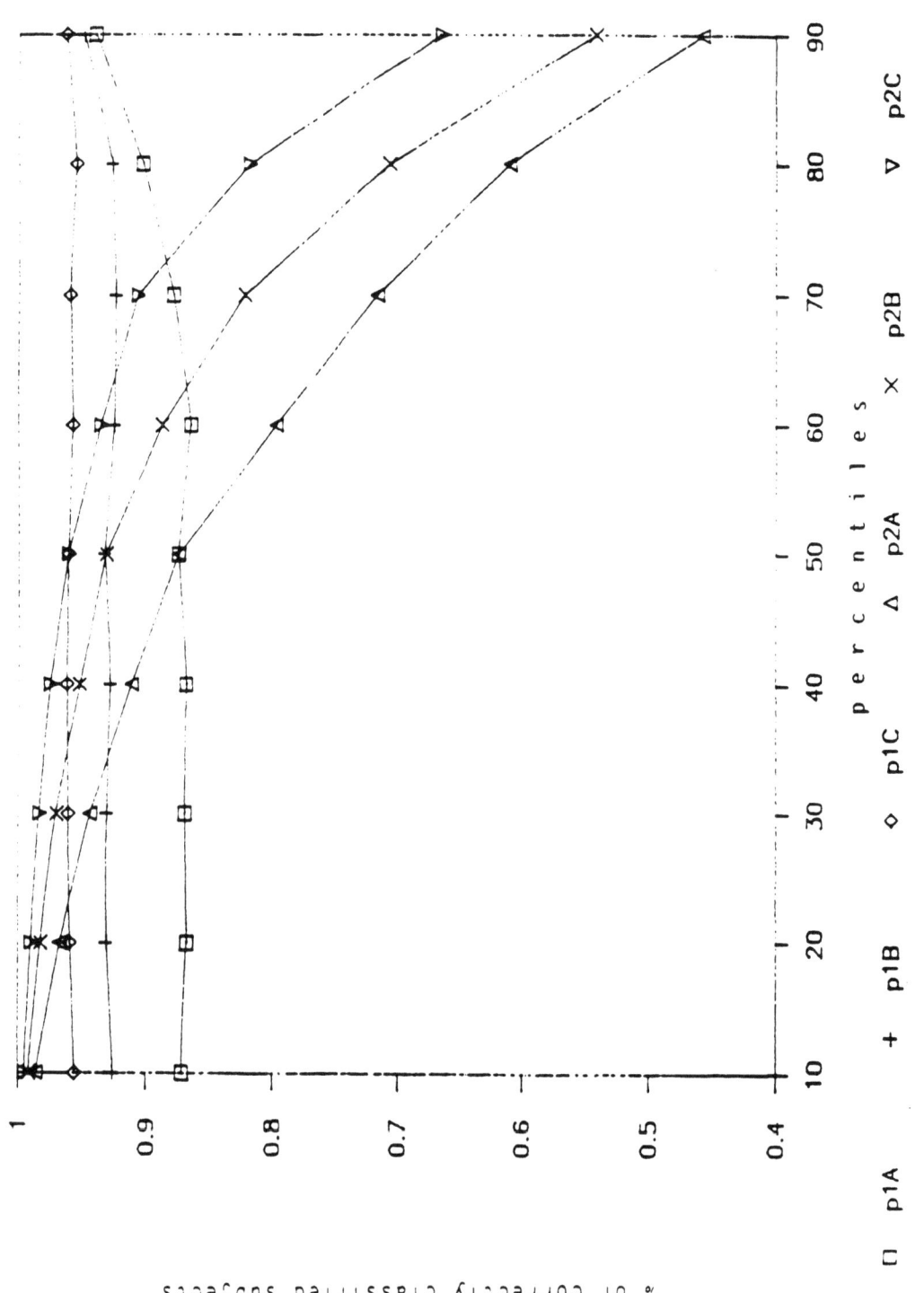

Figure 2

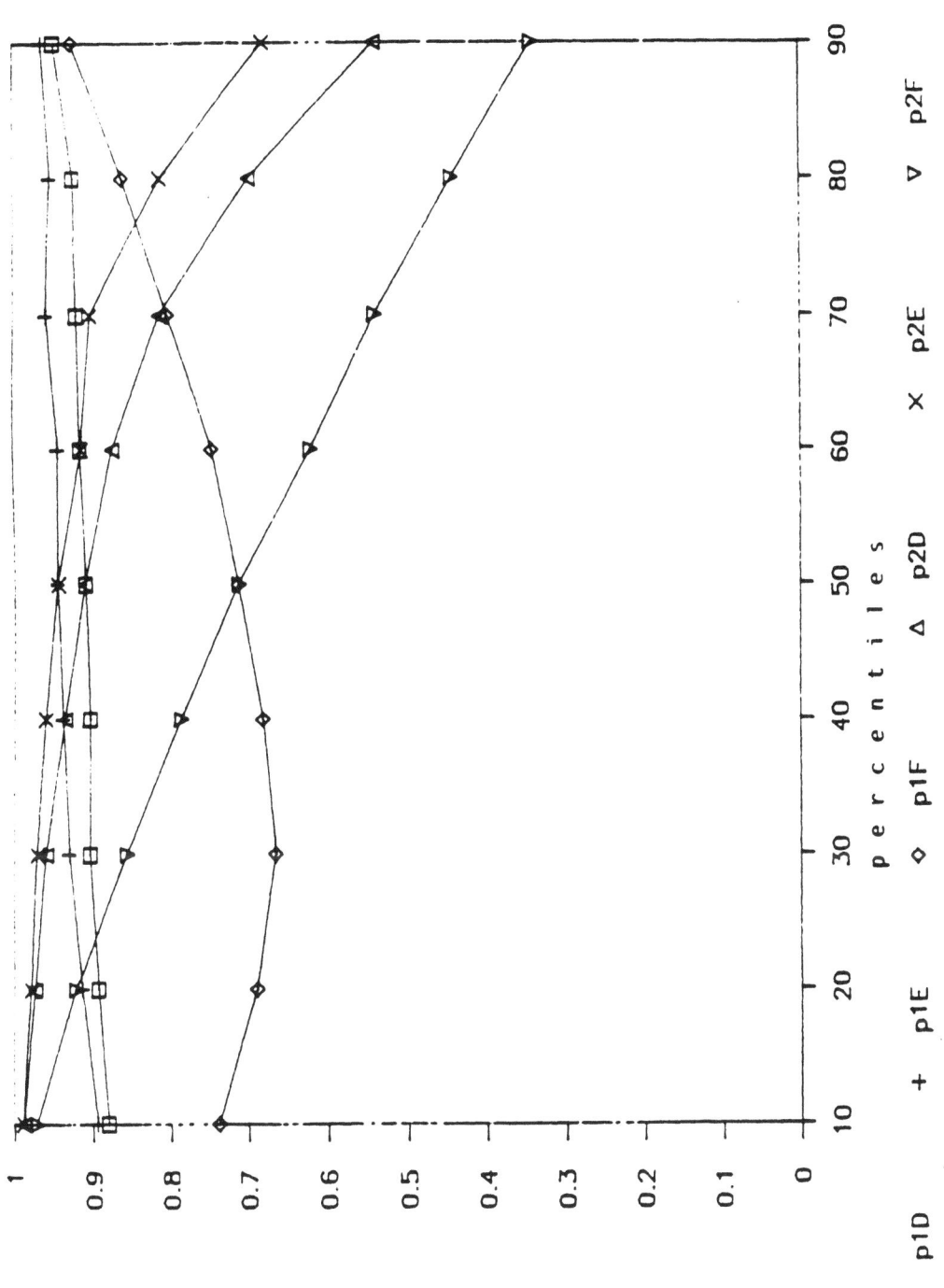

figure 3

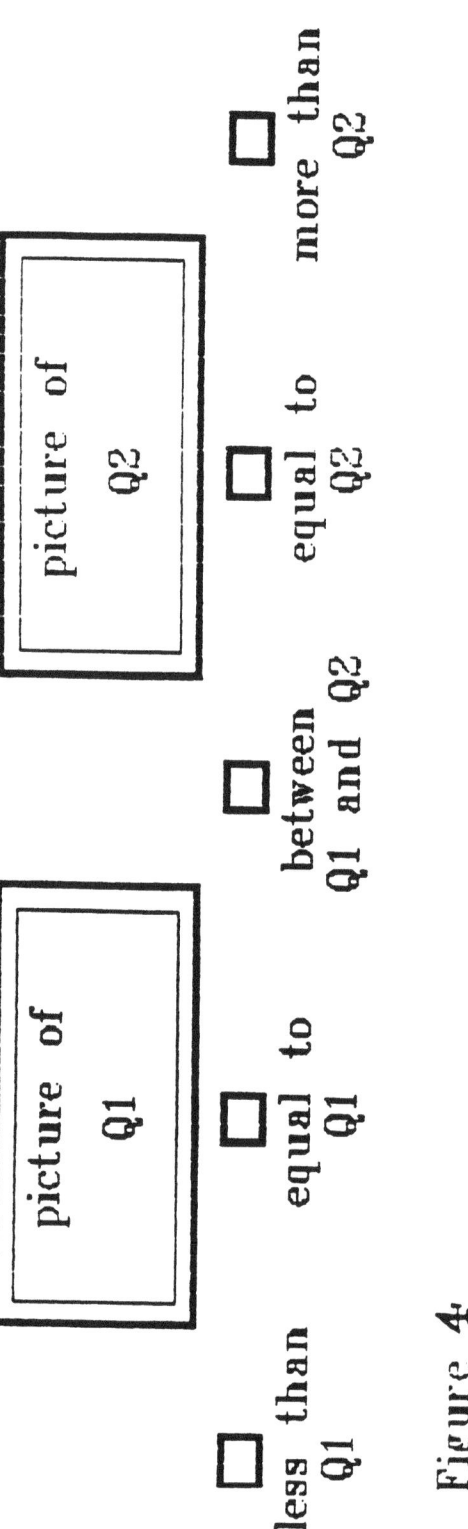

Figure 4

SECTION III

Biochemical, Anthropometric and Other Objective Measures of Diet and Nutritional Status

BIOCHEMICAL INDICATORS OF FAT INTAKE AND THE RISK OF CARDIOVASCULAR DISEASE

S. Renaud[1] & J.L. Martin[2]

[1] INSERM, Unit 63, 22 avenue Doyen Lepine, 69500 Bron, France

[2] INSERM, Unit 265, 151 cours Albert Thomas, 69003 Lyon, France

The role of dietary fat in the pathogenesis of certain diseases has been studied mostly in relation to coronary heart disease (CHD). The main prospective study which has examined the relationship between dietary habits and CHD concluded both after five (Keys, 1970) and after ten years' (Keys, 1980) follow-up that the intake of saturated fat was the leading environmental factor associated with CHD. The mechanism usually put forward to explain the effect of saturated fat in CHD is through the resulting increase in serum cholesterol, particularly LDL cholesterol, and its accumulation in arterial walls. Consequently, serum cholesterol, especially since it can easily be determined, has been considered for half a century to be the main indicator of fat intake as well as the main blood parameter for evaluating the risk of CHD.

Dietary fats are composed of fatty acids which are absorbed in the intestinal tract. Each of these fatty acids has a more or less specific role, certain saturated fatty acids such as myristic and palmitic acids (Keys et al., 1965) being strongly hypercholesterolaemic; others with double bonds in their molecule, especially linoleic acid (2 double bonds), have hypocholesterolaemic effects (Goodnight et al., 1982). These fatty acids can easily be detected in serum or tissues by gas liquid chromatography (GLC), especially now using capillary columns. These fatty acids could be considered to be precise biochemical indicators of fat intake since they are molecules directly absorbed in the gut.

Finally, blood platelets, the main component of a thrombus, which have recently been shown to be involved in unstable angina (Fuster & Chesebro, 1986), have their behaviour markedly well related to the intake of saturated fat as shown by both animal (Renaud & Lecompte, 1970; Renaud et al., 1970) and human (Renaud et al., 1986) studies. They can also be considered to be indicators of fat intake as well as of the risk of CHD since, in an ongoing prospective study in Wales, preliminary analyses of the prevalent cases indicate that in coronary subjects there is a significantly higher response of platelets to aggregation (Yarnell et al., 1987).

The purpose of the present paper is to examine the significance of these different indicators of fat intake in relation to CHD risk.

Serum cholesterol

The relationship between serum cholesterol and the intake of saturated fats has been extensively investigated (Liu et al., 1978). This association was mostly observed in longitudinal studies, cross-sectional designs being apparently not suitable for the study of associations between dietary lipids and blood cholesterol (Jacobs et al., 1979). The lack of associations in cross-sectional studies has been attributed to methodological problems such as limited range of variation in diet within a community, and inter-individual variation in the level of serum cholesterol due to factors other than dietary lipids. Another bias can occur when individuals have modified their diet, switching from high saturated to high polyunsaturated fat due to awareness of hypercholesterolaemia (Liu et al., 1978). Polyunsaturated fatty acids, mostly linoleic acid, are well known to have hypocholesterolaemic effects (Goodnight et al., 1982) while not all saturated fatty acids increase serum cholesterol. Stearic acid (18:0) seems to have no effect, while it is mostly lauric (12:0), myristic (14:0) and palmitic (16:0) acids which are cholesterol-promoting (Keys et al., 1965). Keys et al. reported that changes in serum cholesterol (Δchol) could be predicted by the following formula:

$$\Delta\text{chol} = 1.26 (2 S-P) + 1.5\sqrt{C}$$

in which S is the percentage of calories from saturated fatty acids and C the quantity of dietary cholesterol (in mg/1000 cal/day).

In general serum cholesterol is strongly associated with the intake of saturated fat on a group basis in population studies (Keys, 1970; 1980) but not on an individual basis. This is exactly what we observed in farmers from different regions of France and Great Britain (Renaud et al., 1986). The food intake was carefully assessed by 24 hr recall + weighing of all food consumed over a second 24 hr period + chemical analysis of a duplicate sample of food during that 24 hr period. Evaluating the food intake with these three techniques combined is still probably not ideal since we were covering only two week ys. Nevertheless, in farmers, who take every meal at home and who do not e much change in dietary habits from day to day, it is probably sufficient to characterize individuals. Over a period of three years, 16 groups comprising 360 individuals were evaluated using the same methodology.

Serum cholesterol was significantly positively correlated with the intake of saturated fat ($r = 0.54$, $p < 0.05$), but more significantly inversely correlated with that of the polyunsaturated fatty acids (mostly 18:2) ($r = -0.83$, $p < 0.001$). The more pronounced relationship with 18:2 could be due to the fact that the 16 groups included four groups that had changed diet one and two years before (groups 1 to 4). Excluding these groups, a similar relationship is observed, but it is less significant. This analysis is further explored in Table 1, showing the correlation coefficients on an individual basis in 10 (242 subjects), 12 (284 subjects) and 18 (424 subjects) groups of farmers from France, Great Britain and Belgium. The 242 and 284 subjects do not comprise subjects that have changed diet; they are included in the 424 subjects. These three groups of subjects show basically similar associations, i.e. no significant correlation with the intake of saturated fat, but a highly significant inverse correlation with the intake of 18:2. Calcium (evaluated by chemical analysis of the diet) and 18:3 are slightly inversely correlated with serum cholesterol. The slight inverse correlation is concordant with the slight hypocholesterolaemic effect of calcium. The strong inverse association with 18:2 is somewhat surprising. It is probably due to the fact that some of the population samples we examined, in France and Belgium especially, already had a sizeable intake of 18:2 (6-8% of calories) in comparison to Great Britain (3-4%) as verified by chemical analysis of the duplicate sample of food. In the Seven Country Study, the intake of 18:2 was mostly in the range of 3-4% (Keys, 1970). Under these last conditions, the inverse association with cholesterol could not be observed.

Multivariate analysis of our data, including saturated, mono- and polyunsaturated fatty acids as well as calcium and alcohol on the 424 subjects, shows that serum cholesterol is significantly correlated (inversely) only with 18:2 ($p < 0.0001$) and calcium ($p < 0.005$) (Table 1).

Thus under our conditions the Keys formula does not explain as much as 18:2 and calcium the level of cholesterol. Concerning cholesterol as a risk factor for CHD, it has been well documented in many studies, especially in the recent "MRFIT" study (Martin et al., 1986). Nevertheless, it should be noted that in most of the studies serum cholesterol is an important risk factor when it is above 220 or 240 mg/dl (Keys, 1980; Martin et al., 1986).

Fatty acids

Fatty acids in animal and human tissues may be obtained exogenously from the diet, but a large part of the saturated fatty acids (which are not essential) are synthesized from small molecule precursors. Interconversions can also occur within the body and influence the fatty acid composition of tissue lipids. Other fatty acids can be formed by transformation of dietary fatty acids in such a way that very few fatty acids, when increased in the diet, accumulate as such in tissue lipids (Carroll, 1965) and most of them to no great extent. It has been emphasized that in humans there was a direct mathematical relationship between the average fatty acid composition of the diet and that of subcutaneous adipose tissue (Beynen et al., 1985). Nevertheless, a high correlation coefficient between diet and depot fat was obtained only with polyunsaturated fatty acids but not with mono- or saturated fatty acids. Adipose tissue and plasma phospholipids were analysed before then six months after diet modification in 51 hyperlipidaemic men (Wilson et al., 1971). The intake of saturated fat was decreased from 14.8 (% of calories) to 9.8, and polyunsaturated increased from 5.1 to 15.2 (% of calories). After six months on this diet, myristic acid in adipose tissue had decreased by 28% and that in plasma phospholipids by 16%. However, palmitic acid, the main dietary saturated fatty acid, did not change at all and stearic acid increased by 33% in adipose tissue. Finally, linoleic acid was increased by 15% in adipose tissue and by 14% in plasma phospholipids. Thus, only myristic and linoleic acids showed a pattern in tissues similar to that of diet.

In the 16 groups of farmers classified as in Fig. 1, the main fatty acid composition of plasma total lipids and platelet total phospholipids did not show clear trends as far as 14:0, 16:0, 18:0 and 18:1 were concerned. Multivariate analyses as shown in Table 2 on the 420 subjects between nutrients and the most common fatty acids indicate that 14:0, 16:0 and 18:0 in the platelet phospholipids are not related at all to the intake of saturated fat.

The explanation is that the level of these fatty acids is markedly well regulated by the platelet biosynthesis (Davenas et al., 1984). In contrast, in plasma total lipids there is a slight but significant positive association between the intake of saturated fat and the three main saturated fatty acids mentioned above. The main fatty acid from the diet, at least under the present conditions, which is markedly related to the level of the same fatty acid in plasma and platelet lipids, is 18:2. Nevertheless, its level in plasma and platelets depends also on the proportion of other dietary fatty acids as well as alcohol which seems to have inhibitory effects. Finally, the only fatty acid from platelet phospholipids which is significantly positively related to the intake of saturated fat was 20:3 (n-9), a minor fatty acid derived from 18:0 by saturation and elongation (Holman et al., 1979) considered to be the marker of essential fatty acid deficiency. Although none of the subjects studied were deficient in 18:2, the results indicate that both in plasma and platelets (as illustrated in Fig. 1), on a group or an individual basis, 20:3 (n-9) is highly significantly positively related to the intake of saturated fat (more so than cholesterol) and inversely related to that of 18:2. The interest of 20:3 (n-9) is that a high level of this fatty acid in plasma cholesterol esters (Kingsbury et al., 1974) and in platelet phospholipids (R.A. Riemersma, D. Wood, M. Oliver, Edinburgh, Scotland, personal communications) has been associated with myocardial infarction. Of additional interest is the fact that platelets enriched in 20:3 (n-9) present a hyperaggregability through the production of a monohydroxy derivative via the lipoxygenase pathway (Lagarde et al., 1985). Although further studies are needed to confirm this hypothesis, it seems that 20:3 (n-9) is not only a marker of the intake of saturated fat, but also a substance associated with an increased risk of CHD.

In conclusion, the level of fatty acids in tissues and plasma lipids depends on several dietary parameters with complex relationships. Nevertheless, 20:3 (n-9) or 14:0 + 16:0 + 18:0 in plasma lipids are more closely related to the intake of saturated fat than is cholesterol. The ratio of 18:2/14:0 + 16:0 + 18:0 in plasma lipids certainly reflects closely enough the dietary P/S ratio. It is not surprising that in coronary patients the relative concentration of saturated fatty acids was higher, whereas that of linoleic acid was lower in the plasma lipid esters but not in platelets (Boberg et al., 1985).

Blood platelets

In addition to atherosclerosis, thrombosis contributes significantly to CHD. The thrombotic tendency (in both veins and arteris) has been shown in experimental studies (Hornstra, 1974; Gautheron & Renaud, 1972) to be parallel with the dietary saturated fat content (Fig. 2) mainly through an effect on blood platelets (Renaud & Lecompte, 1970; Renaud et al., 1970)

These experimental results have been reproduced recently in rural populations studied in different areas of France and Great Britain (Renaud et al., 1986). The pilot studies performed in France (Renaud et al., 1979) and Great Britain (Renaud et al., 1981) had indicated that the clotting activity of platelets and their response to thrombin-induced aggregation were more closely related than serum cholesterol to the intake of saturated fatty acids.

In areas with a lower mortality rate from CHD, the intake of saturated fat and the platelet function tests were also lower. These early results were confirmed subsequently in smokers from East and West Scotland (Renaud et al., 1985) and in more extensive studies in 250 farmers from nine areas in France and Great Britain (Renaud et al., 1986). The results obtained concerning the clotting activity of platelets are illustrated in Fig. 3.

Although there is a significant inverse correlation between the intake of saturated fatty acids and the F_3-CT, certain groups apparently do not follow the general trend. In Fig. 4, similar results are illustrated, with both dietary calcium and saturated fatty acids being taken into account in a multivariate linear regression analysis. As a result, the correlation coefficient obtained was r = 0.99 and the association can be satisfactorily compared with that of Fig. 2.

While in animal studies it is possible to vary a single dietary component, human studies are more complex. Populations rarely differ by only one factor even if they are all farmers of the same age. Calcium (from food and mostly water) was one dietary component which was markedly different in the various areas, ranging from 800 to 1400 mg/day.

In man, calcium is known to bind to saturated fatty acids, forming insoluble soaps, which are excreted in the faeces. In animal studies we have also shown similar results with a marked improvement on platelet functions (clotting and thrombin aggregation) (Renaud et al., 1983).

Of interest is the fact that calcium is the main mineral responsible for water hardness. Moreover, regions with hard water have been shown in many countries to have a lower mortality rate from CHD without a satisfactory explanation for the mechanism involved.

The same relationship with saturated fatty acids and calcium has been observed with thrombin-induced aggregation in the nine groups of farmers (Renaud et al., 1986). Finally, it is also of interest that those significant correlations were observed on an individual basis in the 260 subjects as shown in Table 3.

Thus, certain platelet function tests, such as their clotting activity or the response to thrombin aggregation both in animal and human studies, are closely related to the intake of sturated fat, on a group as well as on an individual basis. The effect of saturated fat appears to be regulated by dietary calcium and by 18:3 (linolenic acid, a (n-3) fatty acid precursor of eicosapentaenoic acid) both having possible protective effects on CHD (Goodnight, 1982). Therefore, certain platelet function tests can also be considered to be markers of the intake of saturated fats as well as of other environmental factors involved in CHD. They can also be considered as a means to assess the risk of CHD as suggested recently by a case-control study (Boberg et al., 1985) as well as by a preliminary analysis of prevalent cases of CHD in an ongoing prospective study in Wales (Yarnell et al., 1987).

REFERENCES

Beynen, A.C., Hermus, R.J.J. & Hautvast, J.G.A.J. (1985) A mathematical relationship between the fatty acid composition of the diet and that of the adipose tissue in man. Am. J. Clin. Nutr., 33, 81-85

Boberg, M., Vessby, B. & Croon, L.B. (1985) Fatty acid composition of platelets and of plasma lipid esters in relation to platelet function in patients with ischaemic heart disease. Atherosclerosis, 58, 49-63

Carroll, K.K. (1965) Dietary fat and the fatty acid composition of tissue lipids. J. Am. Oil Chemists Soc., 42, 516-528

Davenas, E., Ciavatti, M., Nordoy, A. & Renaud, S. (1984) Effects of dietary lipids on behaviour, lipid biosynthesis and lipid composition, in rat platelets. Biochim. Biophys. Acta, 793, 278-286

Fuster, V. & Chesebro, J.H. (1986) Mechanisms of unstable angina. N. Engl. J. Med., 315, 1023-1025

Gautheron, P. & Renaud, S. (1972) Hyperlipemia induced hypercoagulable state in rat. Role of an increased activity of platelet phosphatidylserine in response to certain dietary fatty acids. Thromb. Res., 1, 353-370

Goodnight, S.H., Harris, W.S., Connor, W.E. & Illingworth, D.R. (1982) Polyunsaturated fatty acids, hyperlipidemia and thrombosis. Artheriosclerosis, 2, 87-113

Holman, R.T., Smythe, L. & Johnson, B. (1979) Effect of sex and age on fatty acid composition of human serum lipids. Am. J. Clin. Nutr., 32, 2390-2399

Hornstra, G. (1974) Dietary fats and arterial thrombosis. Haemostasis, 2, 21-52

Jacobs, D.R., Jr., Anderson, J.T. & Blackburn, H. (1979) Diet and serum cholesterol: do zero correlations negate the relationship? Am. J. Epidemiol., 110, 77-87

Keys, A. (1970) Coronary heart disease in seven countries. Circulation, 41 (Suppl. 1)

Keys, A. (1980) Seven countries. A multivariate analysis of death and coronary heart disease. Cambridge, Massachusetts, Harvard University Press

Keys, A., Anderson, J.T. & Grande, F. (1965) Serum cholesterol response to changes in the diet. Metabolism, 14, 747-787

Kingsbury, K.J., Brett, C., Stovold, R., Chapman, A., Anderson, J. & Morgan, D.M. (1974) Abnormal fatty acid composition and human atherosclerosis. Postgrad. Med. J., 50, 425-440

Lagarde, M., Burtin, M., Rigaud, M., Sprecher, H., Dechavanne, M. & Renaud, S. (1985) Prostaglandin E_2-like activity of 20:3 (n-9) platelet lipoxygenase end-product. FEBS Lett., 181, 53-56.

Liu, K., Stamler, J., Dyer, A., McKeever, J. & McKeever, P. (1978) Statistical methods to assess and minimize the role of intra-individual variability in obscuring the relationship between dietary lipids and serum cholesterol. J. Chron. Dis., 31, 399-418

Martin, M.J., Hulley, S.B., Browner, W.S., Kuller, L.H. & Wentworth, D. (1986) Serum cholesterol, blood pressure and mortality: implications from a cohort of 361,662 men. Lancet, ii, 933-936

Renaud, S. & Lecompte, F. (1970) Hypercoagulability induced by hyperlipemia in rat, rabbit and man. Role of platelet factor 3. Circulat. Res., 27, 1003-1011

Renaud, S., Kuba, K., Goulet, C., Lemire, Y. & Allard, C. (1970) Relationship between fatty acid composition of platelets and platelet aggregation in rat and man. Relation to thrombosis. Circulat. Res., 26, 553-564

Renaud, S., Dumont, E., Godsey, F., Suplisson, A. & Thevenon C. (1979) Platelet functions in relation to dietary fats in farmers from two regions of France. Thromb. Haemost., 40, 518-531

Renaud, S., Morazain, R., Godsey, F., Dumont, E., Symington, I.S., Gillanders, E.M. & O'Brien, J.R. (1981) Platelet functions in relation to diet and serum lipids in British farmers. Brit. Heart J., 46, 561-570

Renaud, S. Ciavatti, M., Thevenon, C. & Ripoll, J.P. (1983) Protective effects of dietary calcium and magnesium on platelet function and atherosclerosis in rabbits fed saturated fat. Atherosclerosis, 47, 187-198

Renaud, S., Dumont, E., Baudier, F., Ortchanian, E. & Symington, I.S. (1985) Effect of smoking and dietary saturated fats on platelet functions in Scottish farmers. Cardiovasc. Res., 19, 155-159

Renaud, S., Morazain, R., Godsey, F., Dumont, E., Thevenon, C., Martin, J.L. & Mendy, F. (1986) Nutrients, platelet function and composition in nine groups of French and British farmers. Atherosclerosis, 60, 37-48

Wilson, W.S., Hulley, S.B., Burrows, M.I., & Nichaman, M.Z. (1971) Serial lipid and lipoprotein responses to the American Heart Association fat-controlled diet. Am. J. Med., 51, 491-503

Yarnell, J.W.G., Elwood, P.C. & Renaud, S. (1987) Platelet function and ischaemic heart disease in the Caerphilly study. In: Somogyi, J.C., Renaud, S. & Astier-Dumas, M., eds, Emerging Problems in Human Nutrition. Bibliotheca Nutr. Dieta, 40, 10-27

Table 1. Correlation coefficients between serum cholesterol and nutrient intake in French, British and Belgian farmers

Diet	No. of subjects		
	242	284	424
Fatty acids:			
Saturated	0.10	0.00	0.08
Monounsaturated	-0.04	-0.09	-0.08
(18:2)	-0.29***	-0.24**	-0.26***
Linoleic			
(18:3)	-0.16*	0.02	-0.11*
Linolenic			
Calcium	-0.11	-0.08	-0.11*

*p < 0.05
**p < 0.01
***p < 0.0001

Table 2. Stepwise multivariate regression analysis of diet (chemical analysis) and platelet phospholipid fatty acids (and plasma total lipids) in 420 farmers

	14:0	16:0	18:0	18:1	18:2	20:3 (n-9)	20:4 (n-6)
Fatty acids:							
Saturated	–	–	–	–	–	0.26***	0.11*
	(0.13)*	(0.19)***	(0.17)**		(-0.14)**	(0.25)***	(-0.32)****
Monounsaturated	–	–	–	–	–	–	0.11*
	(-0.17)**			(0.13)*			(0.24)****
(18:2) Linoleic	–	–	0.31****	–	0.31****	-0.26****	–
			(0.12)	(-0.53)****	(0.49)****	(-0.39)****	(0.22)****
(18:3) Linolenic	-0.11*	–	-0.14**	–	0.19****	–	-0.11*
							(-0.19)**
Alcohol	–	0.13**	–	–	-0.24****	0.14**	–
		(0.29)***		(0.17)**	(0.27)****		

*p < 0.05
**p < 0.01
***p < 0.001
****p < 0.0001
Standard partial coefficients

In brackets, coefficients for plasma total lipids

Table 3. Multiple regression in 250 French and British farmers between nutrients (chemical analysis) and platelet function tests

	F_3-CT	Thrombin-induced aggregation
Saturated fatty acids	0.46***	0.21***
(18:3) Linolenic	-0.26***	-0.30***
Calcium	-0.22***	-0.15*

*p < 0.05
***p < 0.0001
Standard partial coefficients

The nutrients listed in the Table were the only dietary components determined that were significantly related to the platelet function tests

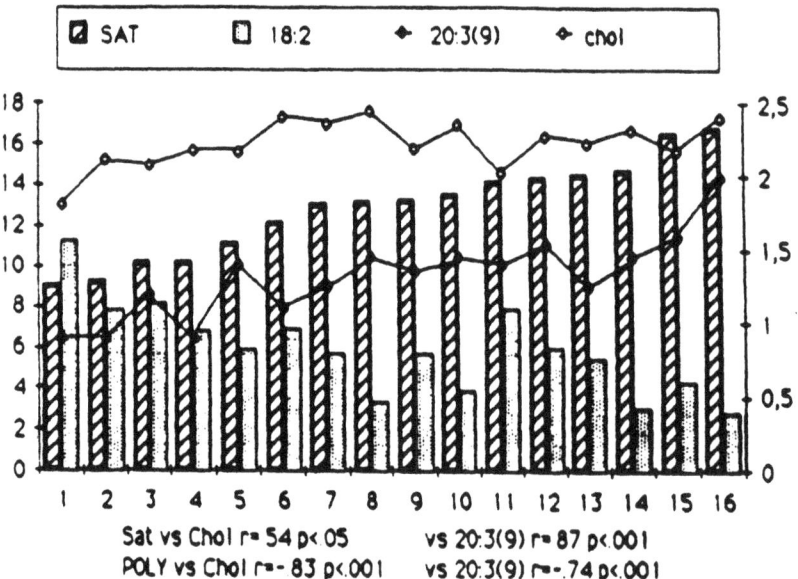

Fig. 1. Sixteen groups of 20 to 42 French and British farmers from different regions, classified according to their intake of saturated (SAT) fats (in % calories from 9 to 17 left scale). Also shown is the intake of 18:2 (% calories), the level of serum cholesterol (chol) (in g/l from 1.8 to 2.4; right scale) and of 20:3(n-9) in platelet phospholipids (from 0.18 to 0.40 %, scale not shown).

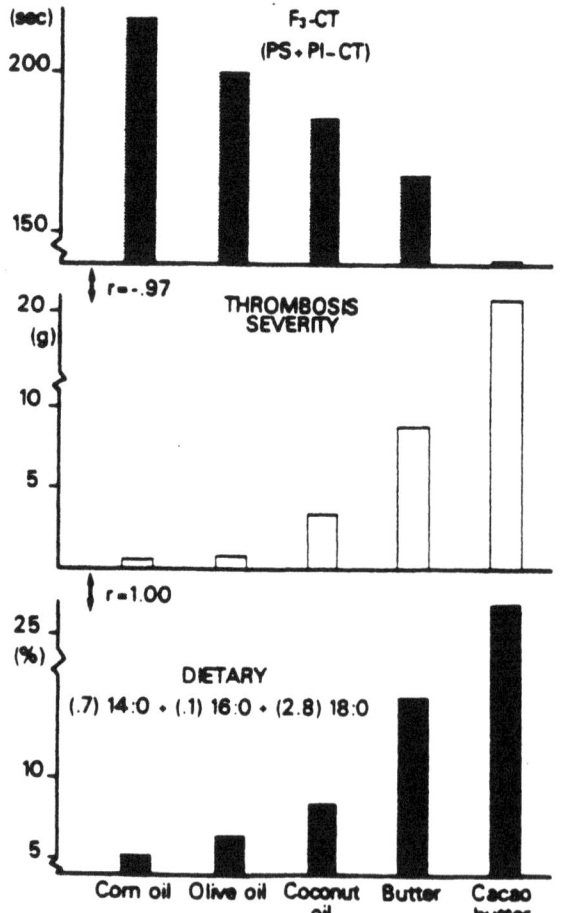

Fig. 2. Relationship between the percentage of 14:0, 16:0 and 18:0 supplied by the diet, the severity of thrombosis and the clotting activity of platelet phospholipid fractions PS + PI or factor 3 clotting activity (F_3-CT). Adapted from Gautheron and Renaud (23) courtesy of Thrombosis Research.

SECTION IV

Prospective Studies on Cancer in Relation to Endogenous and Exogenous Hormones

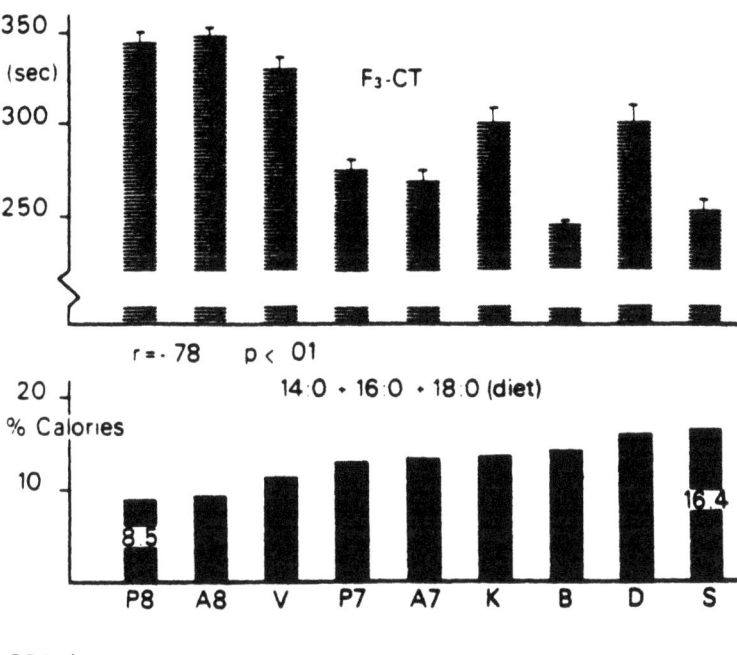

Fig. 3. Nine groups of French and British farmers studied over a period of two years, classified by increasing order according to their intake of saturated fatty acids (14:0 + 16:0 + 18:0) (bottom). At the top of the Figure is shown the corresponding clotting activity of the whole platelets (F_3-CT). Adapted from Renaud et al (8). Courtesy of Atherosclerosis.

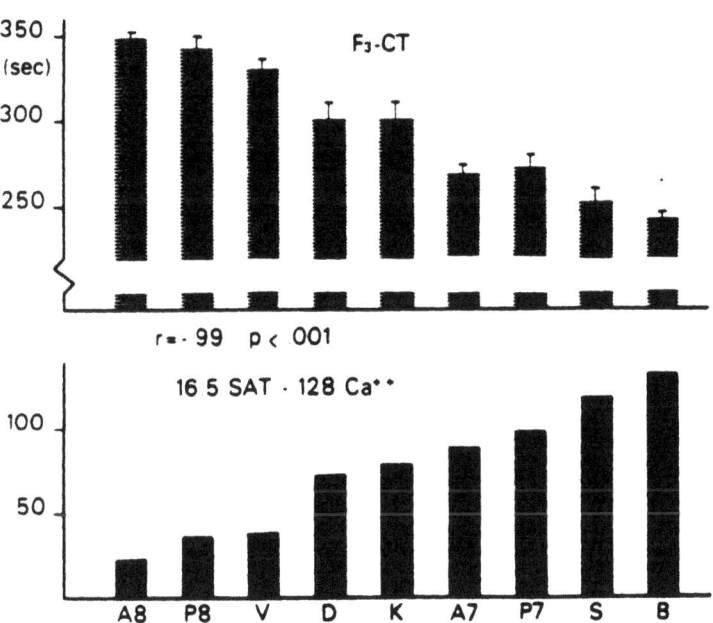

Fig. 4. The nine groups of French and British farmers from Figure 4 classified according to their intake of saturated fat adjusted for their calcium intake (multivariate analysis). Adapted from Renaud et al (8). Courtesy of Atherosclerosis.

CALORIC RESTRICTION IN EARLY LIFE; EFFECTS ON BREAST CANCER RISK FACTORS?

(THE DOM BASED DUTCH FAMINE STUDY)

P.A.H. van Noord[1], H.J.A. Collette[1], F. de Waard[2], J.J. Rombach[1]

[1] Preventicon Rijksuniversiteit Utrecht, Postbus 19006, 3501 DA Utrecht, The Netherlands

[2] Rijksinstitut voor de Volksgezondheid, Postbus 1, 3720 BA Bilthoven, The Netherlands

INTRODUCTION

Caloric restriction has been used since early in this century to slow down maturation speed in rodents (Osborne & Mendel, 1917). In postweaning rodents this led to increased lifespan (Ball et al., 1947). The extension of lifespan was related to decrease and/or postponement of the occurrence of hormone-dependent tumours. Correlated (or possibly mediating) effects described are persistently decreased body weight in deprived animals, altered body proportions (McCay et al., 1935; McCance, 1964) and shifts in indicators of sexual maturation (Merry & Holehan, 1979), menopause (Ball et al., 1947) and fertile periods (Osborn & Mendel, 1917; Kennedy & Mitra, 1963; Dickerson et al., 1964; Glass et al., 1976). However, whether caloric deprivation on life-time cancer risk points towards the role of body weight per se or reflects influences on maturation speed and/or metabolic rate still remains an open question.

Tannenbaum (1945) extended the early experiments to see whether specific components in the calorie-restricted diets (fat versus carbohydrates) produced different effects on this reduction of spontaneous mammary tumours. The group of Ross and Bras (1971) was started in 1950 and, with their isocaloric diet, focused more on the proportion of proteins and the different time windows of vulnerability to caloric restriction in the life of rats. All restricted diets were sufficient in vitamins and other micronutrients in order to ensure that these diets really differed only in their caloric value. Experiments were also carried out with self-selected diets which were different in caloric value so as to make the model best comparable with the dietary situation in humans (Ross et al., 1982). It was found that the ways in which rats metabolized their diets in terms of growth efficiency and "metabolic rate" were the relevant components in a multiple regression model to explain the differences in longevity.

Extrapolation of results from rodents, (rats in particular), however, poses some specific problems. To begin with, at birth a human baby is much more mature than a new-born rat. The life of a rat is measured in weeks, as are the different phases in its life. This makes it rather difficult to translate periods in a rodent's life to comparable phases in human development. Objective signs of sexual maturation in rodents, such as vaginal opening, oestrus and mating behaviour, on which effects of restriction have been shown (Kennedy & Mitra, 1963), are difficult to transpose to stages in human puberty, a comparable relevant time window for possible effects on breast cancer risk initialization.

As far as body proportions are concerned, a study giving data on body length in rodents measured nose to tail distances, which are more or less comparable to the enchondral growth of the human lumbar column. However, most pathways described regarding the nutrition of humans and its effects on hormones relate to the epiphyses of long bones. In humans these are permanently closed at the end of puberty. In the rat, however, the epiphyses only go into a period of quiescence (Silberberg & Silberberg, 1955); they can later be reactivated by somatomedin. Thus, in principle, the rat is able to catch up on growth throughout its life, whereas in humans this is only possible until the end of puberty.

In studies carried out on pigs it was not possible to draw clear-cut conclusions relevant to human skeletal growth (Dickerson et al., 1964; McCance, 1964).

STUDIES OF CALORIC RESTRICTION IN HUMANS

Most global ecological studies correlating breast cancer mortality with per capita fat intake or beef (protein intake) (Wynder et al., 1986) might also be interpreted as a reflection of underlying differences in caloric intake or for that matter caloric expenditure (Willett, 1987) given the results of animal experiments (Kritchevsky et al., 1986).

On the level of human individuals, clinical effects of caloric restriction have been described in anorexia nervosa and chronic diseases (Keys et al., 1950a,b). For prepubertal girls a critical body weight has been postulated by Frisch (1971). Increased calorie expenditure effects have been described among athletes and ballet dancers affecting somatic maturation and hormonal efficiency as reflected in shifts in age of menarche, cycle regularity, and body height and weight for a given age (Frisch et al., 1980, 1981) as well as a decrease in reproductive cancers (Frisch et al., 1985). Starvation itself can lead to a situation described as pseudohypophysectomy (Mulinoz & Pomerantz, 1940). These effects induced by caloric deprivation do seem to relate to known breast cancer risk factors, as they appear to affect breast development, age at menarche, overweight, fertility-related age at first birth, etc. (Sydenham, 1946; Salter et al., 1947; Frisch et al., 1985). However, some of the observational studies in humans might be influenced by mechanisms of self selection of specific types of women who become involved in dancing and athletics, or they may represent selective survival in studies of populations exposed to chronic malnutrition.

Studies have been carried out addressing the anthropometric characteristics of women with and without breast cancer, not the determinants of growth and maturation itself. A study considering most body proportions, bearing in mind what has been described for rodents, has been carried out by Brinkley et al. (1971). Univariate differences in sitting height and body proportions were presented. Most of these effects in the discriminant function reached significance when corrected for the huge differences in the age of cases and controls.

In Western countries, there has been a secular trend towards increasing height, at least at puberty (van Wieringen, 1979), and a steady lowering since 1830 of age at menarche. This has been ascribed to an improvement in the Western diet, both in calories and otherwise (Tanner, 1962; Roberts & Dann, 1975; Warren, 1980; Wysack & Frisch, 1982).

REQUIREMENTS FOR A "QUASI EXPERIMENT" IN HUMANS: THE DUTCH FAMINE AS AN EXAMPLE

An ideal design that could match animal experiments would require a cohort which involuntarily underwent severe caloric deprivation but whose diet was not grossly deficient in essential micronutrients, and a control group differing only in access to sufficient calories. Famines which occurred in several countries during or after the Second World War might be relevant in this perspective. Famines have been documented in the literature in Russia, Greece, Germany, The Netherlands, POW camps and Japan, among others (Burger, 1945; Tannenbaum, 1945; Valaoras, 1946; Keys et al., 1950a, b; Takahashi, 1966).

The Dutch famine of 1944-45 has previously been studied (Stein et al., 1975) to determine persistent effects on brain development, foetal growth (Susser, 1982) and on male body weight (Ravelli et al., 1976). This famine was very well documented compared to other war-related famines. Information is available on the geographical area exposed, documented calorie intake by government food rationing, mortality figures and reports by research and relief teams that visited the area directly after the famine (Burger, 1945; Stare, 1945; Tauber, 1945; Smith, 1947). The Dutch Famine, therefore, comes close to an "experimental design".

A famine combined with a fierce winter struck part of the unliberated western part of the Netherlands between November 1944 and May 1945. Mortality was high, especially among elderly men. After the war the level of food and health care was soon restored to pre-war levels (Dols & Arcken, 1946).

Food rationing had already started in 1939 in anticipation of a long period of neutrality as in 1914-18. This effectively imposed a more uniform pattern of available diet and nutrients throughout the Netherlands during the first four years of the war than in the pre- and post-war situation (Trienekens, 1985). Thus, when the famine actually occurred, food distribution was well established and the rations provided represented caloric intake in the western part of the Netherlands (Fig. 1). During the famine period few cases of specific deficiency syndromes were recorded (such as beriberi or scurvy) although hunger oedema was found. The situation in the famine-exposed area also led to increased caloric requirements due to higher levels of caloric expenditure. No public transport was operational and bicycles, the national means of transportation, were confiscated by the army. By Dutch standards, the winter of 1945 was severe and there was a shortage of fuel for heating and cooking. The clothing scarcity also caused increased calorie requirements in order to maintain body temperature. People, women and older males in particular, made long marches, "hongertochten" to obtain food in farming areas in the eastern part of the Netherlands.

Stress should be mentioned as, in addition to the food shortage, there was the constant threat of air raids and bombardments. This may help to explain effects on women during the war, such as amenorrhea, which might not be soley due to caloric deficiency (Sydenham, 1946).

This Dutch famine can be seen to be an "unnatural" experiment where the effects of self-selection were reduced, and a control population was created in the unexposed, liberated southern and eastern parts of the country, where food was available but could not be transported to the western part because of the blockade.

SOME INDICATIVE RESULTS OF THE DOM PROJECT

The town and province of Utrecht and the two provinces of Holland were in the famine-exposed area. Since 1974 the DOM Project on early breast cancer screening has been operating in Utrecht and its suburbs (de Waard et al., 1984). When comparing the different breast cancers detected by screening, a substantial difference in pick-up rates was found (Table 1) that could not be explained by differences in the cohorts or drift in diagnostic procedures (Rombach, 1986). An alternative explanation was considered, i.e. a persistent effect of the Dutch famine. It must be stressed that at the time of screening not all the women participating had been exposed to the famine. Through migration, women from non-exposed areas have moved to Utrecht thereby diluting, if anything, the possible effect of the famine.

AIMS OF THE STUDY IN THE DOM COHORTS AT UTRECHT

1. Assess the persistency of the effects of the Dutch famine on some risk indicators for (breast) cancer.
2. Assess whether a definite effect on breast cancer itself exists in women, as has been shown to operate in rodents (Table 1).
3. If such an effect exists, assess whether and to what extent such an effect operates through known risk factors, by modifying the relationship between the risk factors and the disease, or by completely independent mechanisms.

Since 1983, women born between 1911 and 1948, who are invited for screening, are asked about their famine exposure. The age range of the women at the time of the famine runs from conception up to 33 years of age. The women filled out a questionnaire to assess famine exposure status, and to assess "intermediate outcomes" (breast cancer risk indicators) such as age at menarche and, if applicable, age at menopause, age at first birth, and perceived fertility. Upon screening, mammography and biometry were performed to measure total body length, weight, sitting height, armspan index and, since 1984, waist and hip girth. Biological material was collected for the purpose of future studies, and the samples stored in a biological bank.

All women in the Utrecht area eligible for screening are followed up for occurrence of breast cancer, whether they actually participated or not. By mid-1987, we plan to have information on approximately 30 000 women who will constitute the cohort to be followed. In due time, possible effects on diseases other than breast cancer will also be investigated.

ACKNOWLEDGEMENTS

This project is funded by the Netherlands Cancer Society KWF (Proj. No. UUKC 85-13).

REFERENCES

Ball, Z.B., Barnes, R.H. & Visscher, M.B. (1947) The effects of dietary caloric restriction on maturity and senescence with particular reference to fertility and longevity. Am. J. Physiol., 150, 511-519

Brinkley, D., Carpenter, R.G. & Haybittle, J.L. (1971) An anthropometric study of women with cancer. Br. J. Prev. Soc. Med., 25, 65-75

Burger, G.C.E. (1943) Starvation in Western Holland. Lancet, i, 282-283

Dickerson, J.W.T., Gresham, G.A. & McCance, R.A. (1964) The effect of undernutrition and rehabilitation on the development of the reproductive organs in pigs. J. Endocrinol., 29, 111-118

Dols M.J.L. & Arcken, D.J.A.M. (1946) Food supply and nutrition in the Netherlands during and immediately after World War II. Millbank Mem. Fund Quart., 24, 319-358

Frisch, R.E. (1971) Height and weight at menarche and a hypothesis of critical body weights and adolescent events. Science, 169, 397-399

Frisch, R.E., Wyshak, G. & Vincent, L. (1980) Delayed menarche and amenorrhea in ballet dancers. New Engl. J. Med., 303, 17-19

Frisch, R.E., von Gotz-Welbergen, A.V., McArthur, J.W. et al. (1981) Delayed menarche and amenorrhea of college athletes in relation to age of onset of training. J. Am. Med. Assoc., 246, 1559-1563

Frisch, R.E., Wysach, G., Albright, N.L. et al. (1985) Lower prevalence of breast cancer and cancers of the reproductive system among former college athletes compared to non athletes. Br. J. Cancer, 52, 885-891

Glass, A.R., Harrison, R. & Swerdloff, R.S. (1976) Effects of undernutrition and amino acid deficiencies on the timing of puberty in the rat. Pediatr. Res., 10, 951-955.

Kennedy, G.C. & Mitra, J. (1963) Body weight and food intake as initiating factors for puberty in the rat. J. Physiol., 166, 408-418

Keys, A. et al. (1950a) The history of starvation. In: The biology of human starvation, Vol. 1, Chapter 1

Keys, A. et al. (1950b) Anorexia nervosa and pituitary cachexia. In: The Biology of Human Starvation, Vol. 2, Chapter 44

Kritchevsky, D., Weber, M.M., Buck, C.L. & Klurfeld, D.M. (1986) Calories, fat and cancer. Lipids, 21, 222-284

McCance, R.A. (1964) Some effects of undernutrition. J. Pediatr., 65, 1008-1014

McCay, C.M., Crowell, M.F. & Maynard, L.A. (1935) The effect of retarded growth on length of lifespan and upon the ultimate body size. J. Nutr., 10, 63-79

Merry, B.J. & Holehan, A.N. (1979) Onset of puberty and duration of fertility in rats fed a restricted diet. J. Reprod. Fertil., 57, 253-259

Mulinoz, M.G. & Pomeranz, L. (1940) Pseudo hypophysectomy. A condition resembling hypophysectomy produced by malnutrition. J. Nutr., 19, 493-504

Osborne, T.B. & Mendel, F.E.L. (1917) The effect of retardation of growth upon breeding period and duration of life of rats. Science, 45, 294

Ravelli, G.P., Stein, Z. & Susser, M. (1976) Obesity in young men after famine exposure in utero and early infancy. New Engl. J. Med., 295, 349-353

Roberts, D.F. & Dann, T.C. (1975) A 12 year study of menarcheal age. Br. J. Prev. Soc. Med., 29, 31-39

Rombach, J.J. (1986) Diagnostische Beschouwingen 59-85. In: Het DOM Project voor de Vroege Opsporing van Borstkanker te Utrecht, Vol. III, Chapter VI

Ross, M.H. & Bras, G. (1971) Lasting influence of early caloric restriction on prevalence of neoplasms in the rat. J. natl. Cancer Inst., 47, 1095-1113

Ross, M.H., Lustbader, E.D. & Bras, G. (1982) Dietary practices of early life and spontaneous tumors of the rat. Nutr. Cancer, 3, 150-167

Salter, W.T., Klatskin, G. & Humm, F.D. (1947) Gynaecomastia due to malnutrition. II. Endocrine studies. Am. J. Med. Sci., 213, 31-36

Silberberg, M. & Silberberg, R. (1955) Diet and life span. Physiol. Rev., 35, 347-362

Smith, C. (1947) Effects of maternal undernutrition upon the newborn infants in Holland (1944-1945). J. Pediatr., 30, 229-243

Stare, F.J. (1945) Nutritional conditions in Holland. Nutr. Rev., 3, 225-227

Stein, Z., Susser, M., Saenger, G. & Marolla, F. (1975) Famine and Human Development. The Dutch Hunger Winter of 1944-45. Oxford University Press, Oxford

Susser, M. (1982) Third variable analysis: Application to causal sequences among nutrient intake, maternal weight, birthweight, placental weight and gestation. Statistics in Medicine, 1, 105-120

Takahashi, E. (1966) Growth and environmental factors in Japan. Human Biol., 38, 112-130

Tannenbaum, A. (1945) The dependence of tumor formation on the composition of the calorie-restricted diet as well as on the degree of restriction. Cancer Res., 5, 616-625

Tanner, J.M. (1962) Growth at Adolescence, 2nd Edition, Oxford, Blackwell Scientific Publications, Fig. 53

Trienekens, G.M.T. (1985) Tussen ons Volk en de Honger. De Voedselvoorziening 1940-1945. Utrecht, Diss. RUU.

Tauber, J. (1945) Netherland children in England. Br. Med. J., 6, 486

Valaoras, V.G. (1946) Some effects of famine on the population of Greece. Human Biol., 42, 184-201

de Waard, F., Collette, H.J.A., Rombach, J.J., Baanders-van Halewijn, E.A. & Honing, C. (1984) The DOM project for the early diagnosis of breast cancer. J. Chron. Dis., 37, 1-44

Warren, M.P. (1980) The effects of exercise on pubertal progression and reproductive function in girls. J. Clin. Endocrinol. Metab., 51, 1150-1157

Willett, W.C. (1987) Implications of total energy intake for epidemiologic studies of breast and colon cancer. Am. J. Clin. Nutr., 45, 354-360

van Wieringen, J.C. (1979) Secular growth changes in the Netherlands 1850-1978. Coll. Antropol., 3, 35-47

Wynder, E.L., Rose, D. & Cohen, L. (1986) Diet and breast cancer in causation and therapy. Cancer, 59, 1804-1813

Wysack, G. & Frisch, R.E. (1982) Evidence for a secular trend in age of menarche. New Engl. J. Med., 306, 1033-1035

Table 1. Absolute and relative frequency of breast cancer detected by age among two cohorts (DOM I[a] and DOM II[b]) in the DOM project in Utrecht[c]

Age at screening	Number of women screened		Breast cancers detected			
			Number		Percentage	
	DOM I	DOM II	DOM I	DOM II	DOM I	DOM II
≤ 54	7 125	10 491	43	38	0.60	0.36
55-59	8 107	3 754	43	13	0.53	0.35
≥ 60	8 279	2 287	77	19	0.93	0.83
Total	23 511	16 532	163	70		

[a]DOM I cohort women born 1911-1925 (20-23 years old in 1944-45).

[b]DOM II cohort women born 1917-1931 (14-27 years old in 1944-45)

[c]Data from the first DOM report include all women living in Utrecht and suburbs at the time of the screening (1974-1984). This is not identical to being exposed to the famine in 1944-45).

DIAGRAM

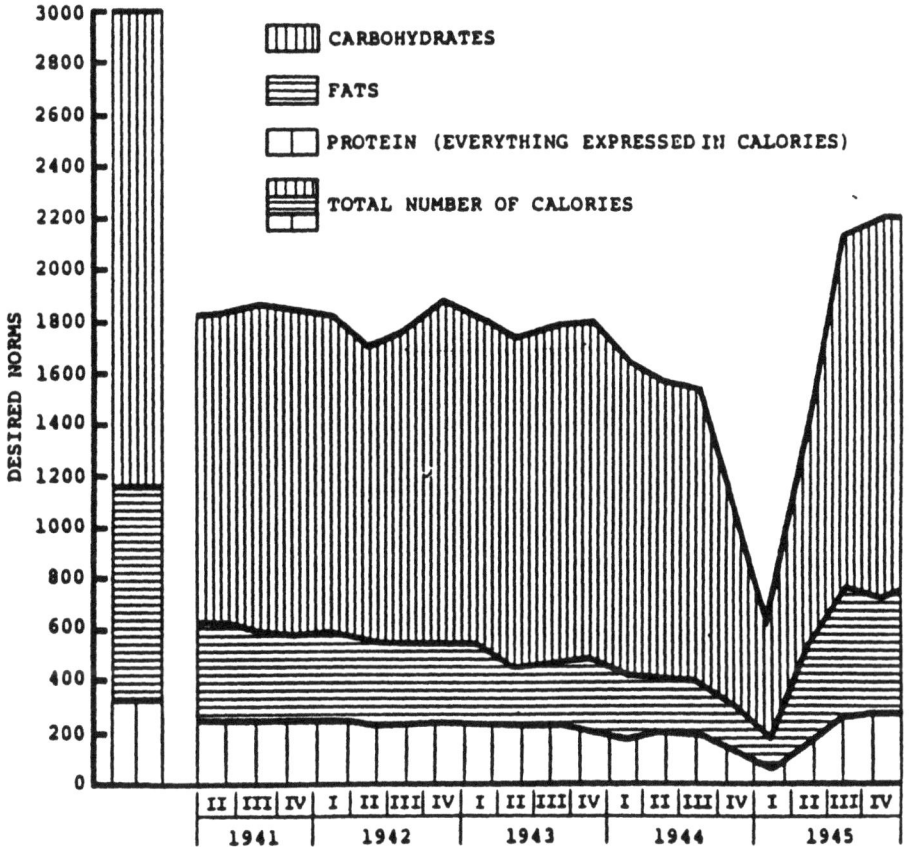

Figure 1. Average quarterly distribution of food rations in Calories, protein, fats, and carbohydrates in the western Netherlands, 1941 through 1945.
Source: Reproduced from Burger, Drummond, and Sandstead, 1948, Part I, p. 6.

ANTHROPOMETRIC MEASUREMENTS IN RELATION TO HORMONAL PATTERNS AND BREAST CANCER

S. Panico

Istituto de Medicina Interna e Malattie Dismetaboliche, 2 'Facolta' di Medicina, Universita di Napoli

Many experimental, clinical and epidemiological observations suggest that body size and structure may influence the development of most chronic diseases. Breast cancer is among these. The relationship between body size and structure and hormonal pattern may be the key to elucidate this influence on breast cancer.

Anthropometric measurements, the way in which body size and structure can be measured, are the general topic of this paper. The main focus, however, is on what can be called "less common" anthropometric measurements — other than height, weight or any relative weight index — and their possible relationship to hormonal patterns and breast cancer risk.

The base for this contribution has been the discussion during the design phase of the ORDET STUDY, a prospective study on the hormonal and nutritional etiology of breast cancer (Berrino et al., 1988). Therefore comments and discussion will be referred essentially to adult women.

We asked ourselves two questions (1) Is there any rationale for looking at these measures rather than height and weight or some common relative weight index? (2) What problems of validity and reproducibility can be raised by using these measurements in epidemiological studies?

On the first question I will try to develop three lines of discussion. Finally some comments will be made on the second question.

1.1 As to anthropometry most information on breast cancer epidemiology is on obesity, which is a measure of body size. Even among some conflicting results, risk due to obesity has been recognized in post-menopausal women. The magnitude of this risk is unable to explain major differences in incidence between different populations, as for many other risk factors for breast cancer. The mechanism suggested for this effect indicates that the adipose tissue play an important role. In fact the main observations in obese individuals are (a) androstenedione production rates are elevated and serve as pre-hormones of both testosterone and oestrogens, (b) peripheral aromatization of androgens to form oestrogens, mainly androstenedione to oestrone, is increased, (c) Sex-Hormone-Binding-Globulin (SHBG) is decreased (Kirschinner et al., 1981).

Since the main metabolic pathways described above take place in the adipose tissue the questions are: Do we need to measure obesity or fatness? Can we use a measure of body size or do we need a measure of body composition, with special reference to the amount of fat? And if the answer is that we have to measure fatness, the other question is: which measure should we take?

Body composition shows up to be more and more informative than body size. Fat is distributed in various regions of the body in different ways. Adipocytes have different size according to their localization and this difference in size determines differences in metabolic functions. For instance, gluteal fat cells are larger than abdominal and these are larger than subscapular. The gluteal fat cells are more sensitive to oestrogens than other regional cells. They are characterized by high levels of lipoproteinlipase compared to the abdominal ones, most pronounced in fertile and pregnant women, less pronounced in post-menopausal women. The hypothesis that can be generated from this is that adipocites in the gluteal fat have specific endogenous characteristics with lipoproteinlipase activity sensitive to endocrine regulation (Rebuffe-Scrive et al., 1985; Clarkson et al., 1980).

Actually this changes the picture of how to measure obesity, how to consider obesity and fatness, body size and body composition, focusing on adipocytes and the different role they can play in different regions of the body.

Therefore measures of regional fat distribution may explain, probably in a better way, the mechanism linking on the one side body fat to obesity and on the other side hormonal patterns and breast cancer risk.

One of the most used measurements of body fat distribution is the waist to hip ration. The use of this measurement has divided up individuals in two groups called "apples" and "pears". Apples are those with a higher waist to hip ratio, showing an android type fat distribution, and pears are those with a lower ration, showing gynoid type fat distribution.

The most common relative weight index is the Quetelet index. It is a classical measure of body size, independent of age, and can also be used as a measure of body fat (Garrow et al., 1985). It has usually a good correlation when compared with estimates of body density, which is a measure of body fat. The accuracy of the Quetelet index, compared to other measures, such as skinfold thickness, is lower even if this difference tends to disappear in massively obese individuals. That means that the Quetelet index has a good level of accuracy in clinical studies on obesity, but is less efficient in epidemiological studies (Garrow et al., 1985; Keys et al., 1972).

Skinfold thickness and arm circumferences taken at various sites enable us to measure and localize body fat. Biceps, triceps, subscapular or suprailiac are the most widely used skin folds. Some index used as measures of body fat include either skinfold only (sum of two or more) or skinfolds and circumferences in specific regions – specific and overall fat areas may be estimated (Himes et al., 1980) –, or even putting together skinfolds, circumferences, weight and height – fat and lean mass may be estimated (Fuchs et al., 1978).

Body fat measures are of slightly different levels of accuracy. In spite of some inconsistencies correlation coefficients deriving from comparison of skinfold thickness and corresponding fat areas with body density (a measure of fatness) may be summarized as follows. The correlation is negative and index of biceps and triceps skinfold measurements together is more accurate than single biceps or triceps skinfold or fat areas measured at a single point in different age groups. Moreover a cumulative index of fat areas is more accurate than homologous skinfold thickness, that means that the more regional measurement you measure the better it is (Himes et al., 1980).

1.2 Two questions are relevant when body composition is considered in epidemiological studies on breast cancer.

The first is: Are measures of body fat and its distribution more predictive for breast cancer than any relative weight index?

The second is: What hormonal patterns are interrelated with body fat and its distribution? We can try to discuss some information to reply to this question.

As to the first question we do not know the answer, because there are no data to answer the question.

As to the second piece of information, it comes from the TOPS Study (Take Off Pounds Sensibly) carried out on more than 50 000 women aged 20-59 (Hartz et al., 1984). Some signs of hormonal disease such as irregular cycles, long cycles, hirsutism are quite well predicted by the waist to hip ratio. In the same study the risk of disease such as hypertension, diabetes and gall-bladder disease or symptoms such as menstrual abnormalities is significantly higher in women with upper body fat predominance compared with women with lower body fat predominance even when adjusted for age and relative weight. The finding of risk excess for menstrual abnormalities still detectable after adjustment is of great interest because in another TOPS report waist to hip ratio is found related to age and overweight degree (Lanska et al., 1985).

Another piece of information has been communicated: SHBG is decreased in android type fat distribution (Bruning et al., 1985). This observation seems to be very important, considering the crucial role that sex hormone binding globulin may play in the balance between androgens and oestrogens on the one side and SHBG bound hormones and free hormones on the other.

The lower fat predominance has been always considered as influenced by oestrogen levels even if population based information is not available. The reverse (that body fat distribution influence hormonal level) is also plausible according to the knowledge that peripheral production of oestrogens from androgens occurring in the adipose tissue, is affected by the aromatase activity which can vary according to the body region.

The overall conclusion is that fat distribution is interrelated with hormonal patterns. But the complicated question to be answered is: is fat distribution dependent on the level of sex hormones? Or the direction of the relation is the other way round? Or both? Android type distribution is associated to menstrual abnormalities not more than other diseases (Hartz et al., 1984). And this suggests that fat distribution may influence hormonal patterns, causing menstrual abnormalities, and not vice versa. Moreover the observation that adipocytes play a major role in the peripheral synthesis of oestrogens from androstenedione and that adipocytes may have different metabolic functions according to site, suggests that the oestrogen synthesis may occur in some adipocytes more than in others. And this influenced by fat distribution type.

1.3 Some insights can be received looking at cardiovascular epidemiology studies.

Results from the cross-sectional TOPS Study suggest that in different categories of obesity there is still a role played by waist to hip ratio in determining the prevalence of hypertension. The same is reported for diabetes. These findings are consistent with other cross sectional observations that confirm that fat distribution is a good indicator of the pattern of cardiovascular risk (Contaldo et al., 1986). In the longitudinal observations from a Swedish study the probability of remaining free of myocardial infarction for the women in the first quintile of the distribution of the waist to hip ratio is lower than for those in the fifth quintile. The same behaviour is reported for the probability of survival for many causes of death and the differences are statistically significant. In the same study a statistically significant positive association between waist to hip ratio and myocardial infarction, stroke and death is found after adjustment for age, body mass index and the three major risk factors (Lapidus et al., 1984).

All these observations point in the same direction: the type of fat distribution is independently associated with a pattern of risk for a chronic disease or with that disease.

2.1 The issue of validity and reproducibility of anthropometric measurements is obviously crucial for epidemiologists and has the same weight as the assertment of a rationale for the use of these measures.

As to the accuracy of skinfold thickness as a measure of fat quantity, it has been shown that in very obese people the fat mass can be underestimated. On the other side of the distribution, the very thin people, these problems of accuracy are less important.

As to the waist to hip ratio there is evidence that women with high values of this ratio have a greater quantity of their fat in the interabdominal deposits than do women with low values. This observation has been made through computer tomography (Ashwell et al., 1985).

As to reproducibility there are differences between the left and the right side of the body for single skinfold measurements, but an integrated index (i.e. sum of all skinfolds) is well reproducible. In women for single sites the best reproducibility is for triceps and subscapular skinfolds, less reproducible are biceps and suprailiac. For all these measurements experienced observers are reported to take higher values than untrained observers. In the reproductive phase of woman life, cyclic hormonal and metabolic activity do not have significant influence on skinfold measurements.

The waist circumference is very sensitive to change in energy intake causing problems of reproducibility for the waist to hip ratio measurements. This may have some implications in case-control studies where measurements in cases can be influenced by the nutritional status due to the disease or its consequences. To measure circumferences is however a very quick procedure. A couple of minutes more are needed to measure skinfolds.

In conclusion, there are indications to implement the use of fat distribution measurements in studies on hormones and breast cancer, even if major attention must be paid to reproductibility problems, through careful standardization of observers and subject conditions. In large cohort studies such measurements may be useful also in the view of possible extension of the analysis to pathology other than cancer such as cardiovascular disease.

REFERENCES

Berrino, F. (This report 1988) Prospective studies on hormones and etiology of breast cancer

Kirschner, M.A. et al. (1981) Obesity, hormones and cancer. Cancer Res., 41: 3711

Rebuffe-Scrive, M. et al. (1985) Fat cell metabolism in different regions in women. J. Clin. Invest., 75: 1973

Clarkson, P.M. et al. (1980) Regional adipose cellularity and reliability of adipose cell size determination. Am. J. Clin. Nutr., 33: 2234

Garrow, J.S. et al. (1985) Quetelet's index as a measure of fatness. Int. J. Obesity 9: 147

Keys, A. et al. (1972) Indices of relative weight and obesity. J. Chron. Dis., 25: 329

Himes, J.H. et al. (1980) Fat areas as estimates of total body fat. Am. J. Clin. Nutr., 33: 2093

Fuchs, R.J. et al. (1978) A nomogram to predict lean body mass in men. Am. J. Clin. Nutr., 31: 673

Hartz, A.J. et al. (1978) The association of girth measurements with disease in 32,856 women. Am. J. Epidemiol., 119: 71

Lanska, D.J. et al. (1985) Factors influencing anatomic location of fat tissue in 52,593 women. Int. J. Obesity, 9: 29

Bruning, P. et al. (1986) Personal communication. Meeting of the European Group on Breast Cancer. S. Margherita Ligure

Contaldo, F. et al. (1986) Body fat distribution and cardiovascular risk in middle age in Southern Italy. Atherosclerosis, 61: 169

Lapidus, N. et al. (1984) Distribution of adipose tissue and risk of cardiovascular disease and death: a 12-year follow-up of participants in the population study of women in Göteborg, Sweden. Br. Med. J., 289: 1257

Ashwell, M. et al. (1985) Obesity: new insight into the anthropometric classification of fat distribution shown by computer tomography. Br. Med. J., 290: 1692

SECTION IV

OVERVIEW OF THE ETIOLOGICAL HYPOTHESES LINKING ENDOGENOUS
STEROID HORMONES AND BREAST CANCER

Berrino F., Muti P. and Pisani P.

Istituto Nazionale per lo Studio e la Cura dei Tumori, Milan, Italy

A dozen hormonal hypotheses have been proposed for breast cancer (B.C.) etiology in the last 30 years. A tentative list is shown in Fig. 1, along with the periods during which they have been actively investigated.

A few of them are out of fashion, others appear to be remarkably tenacious, even in absence of much empirical support.

None of them should be considered definitively falsified. Most of these hypotheses have such a core of biological plausibility and/or empirical evidence that it would be unwise to abandon them just because they seem contradicted by some "fact". In this field most epidemiological studies are afflicted by serious limitations in the design, and sometimes in the analysis. It is hard, therefore, to state what a "fact" is in hormones and B.C.

The aim of this paper is to critically review the empirical evidence linking steroid hormones and B.C., and to discuss such a divergent framework of hormonal theories from an epidemiological perspective.

Many excellent epidemiological and physiological reviews are available (Kirschern 1979; Zumoff 1981;, 1982; Petrakis et al., 1982; Kelsey and Hildreth 1983; Moore et al., 1986a; Miller 1987), however, we will only focus on those aspects that can be addressed by new epidemiological approaches.

BIOCHEMICAL AND PHYSIOLOGICAL BACKGROUND

The interpretation and discussion of hormonal hypotheses and their interrelationship require reference to the main metabolic pathways of sex steroid hormones (Bondy 1985; Yen and Jaffe 1986). These are summarized in Fig. 2. Steroid hormones in females are synthesized either in the ovary or in the adrenal gland, but many other tissues contribute to their metabolism.

The synthesis starts from cholesterol, whose side chain at carbon (C) 17 is cleaved between C 20 and C 22 to give delta 5 pregnenolone. From this substance two metabolic pathways follow: delta 5 and delta 4. They are named according to whether the double bond between the 5th and 6th carbon is shifted or not to carbon 4 and 5, that is from B to A ring. This shift is associated with the oxidation of the 3 beta hydroxyl of cholesterol to a ketone, which is essential for the acquisition of androgenic power.

As shown in Figs. 2 and 3, the delta-5-(3-beta-hydroxy)-delta-4-(3-ketone) shift may occur at any step. When it occurs at the first step, Progesterone (P) is produced. The following reactions lead through a further cleavage of the side chain at C 17 to a family of 17-ketosteroids, from which the major androgens and estrogens derive. These 17-ketosteroids, whose main representatives in blood are dehydroepiandrosterone (DHEA), its sulphate (DHEAS), and androstenedione (Adione), are sometimes called "neutral" to distinguish them from estrone (EI), which is also 17-keto but acid, and "11 deoxy" to distinguish them from the 17-ketosteroids coming from the corticosteroids, which have an oxigen in C 11. They are also named adrenal androgens because they are produced mainly by the adrenals and are slightly androgenic. Apart from being precursors of more active molecules, their role is not known.

The full androgenic activity requires a hydroxyl at carbon 17. The 17-beta hydroxylation of adione produces testosterone (T). Adione and T may be aromatized into estrogens, respectively, into estrone (EI) and estradiol (E2) either in the granulosa cells of the ovarian follicle or in aromatase rich peripheral tissues, such as adipose tissue. Estrogenic activity requires a phenolic structure in A ring.

In Fig. 3 dotted lines indicate the hormonal families to which the hypotheses listed in Fig. 1 refer i.e. the progestogens area, the "adrenal" 17 keto androgens area, the major androgens area, and the estrogens area. Fig. 3 also shows a sex hormone binding globulin (SHBG) area. The most active steroid hormones, in fact, are bound almost entirely to plasma proteins while circulating in the blood. The prevailing interpretation of this is that it prevents diffusion into tissues and rapid clearance. About 66% of T and 36% of E2 is bound to SHBG, whereas 30% and 60%, respectively, is bound to albumin, and 1% and 2%, respectively, is free. Adione, on the contrary, binds mainly to albumin and only about 7% specifically to SHBG. The physiological meaning of steroid-protein interaction, however, is not completely understood (Bradlow 1987). The adrenal gland is capable of forming all known active steroids (Bondy 1985). Among sex hormones it produces mainly 17 ketosteroids, but a large fraction of circulating T also derives from the adrenal, either directly or through peripheral conversion.

Adione and T are produced in the ovary, either via delta 5 or delta 4, mostly by the thecal-interstitial cells, which are analogous to the Leydig cells of male gonad, whereas aromatization occurs in the granulosa compartment of the follicle.

The regulation of follicular maturation and selection of which follicle will ovulate, depends on a complex interrelationship between androgens, estrogens and gonadotropins (Fritz and Speroff 1982). Ovulation will occur in the follicle where an estrogenic microenvironment prevails, after an estrogenic threshold is reached.

Blood quantitations of E2, P, 17 OH-P, adione, and to a lesser extent T, show considerable variations during the menstrual cycle. The lowest ovarian contribution to their secretion, and hence the lowest blood concentrations, occur during the first week of the cycle. Androgens and estrogens show their highest levels during mid-cycle and progestogens during the luteal phase.

Low serum levels of P or urine levels of pregnanediol in the second half of the cycle indicate that ovulation did not take place. Anovulatory cycles are frequent in the postmenarche and premenopause years.

Cycle length depends mostly on the follicular phase, which, in turn, depends on the estrogen levels and particularly on the timing of midfollicular E2 rise. The postovulatory length of the cycle, on the contrary, is much more constant.

In the postmenopausal ovary granulosa cells have disappeared, but interstitial cells continue to produce androgens and are still capable of hypertrophy in response to gonadotropins (Yen and Jaffe 1986). After menopause most estrogens derive from peripheral conversion of adrenal and ovarian adione to E1, mainly in adipose tissue.

STEROID HORMONE HYPOTHESES

The causes of B.C. are not known. We have learned from migrant studies that international differences are mostly due to environmental causes, but no environmental factor has since been identified that is sufficient to explain the differences. B.C. incidence is up to ten times higher in West U.S. in white women, than in rural Japan or in poor developing countries (Waterhouse et al., 1982). To explain such a difference, a risk factor should be associated to a relative risk (RR) higher than 10, and should be over ten times more prevalent in high rather than low risk countries (Breslow and Day 1980). In practice these conditions are much more stringent.

Fig. 4 shows the RR that should be associated to a risk factor in order to explain a ten-fold difference between two countries as a function of the prevalence of the exposure. (To explain a ten-fold international difference in lung cancer incidence, for example, a factor such as tobacco smoking, which concerns about 80% of males in developed countries and is about 50 times less prevalent in developing countries, should increase the incidence 15 times, which is not far from the truth).

The risk factors that have been fairly consistently identified up to now (Kelsey et al., 1983), such as early menarche, late menopause, nulliparity, late first pregnancy, rich diet, obesity, low exercise (Frisch et al., 1985), family history, whether combined or not, are at most associated with a RR of 3, one order of magnitude less than what would be necessary to explain the international differences. One must consider that the strength of the association between a given factor and an illness may be considerably reduced if a study is carried out in countries where only limited range of the distribution (of the values of the factor) can be explored, e.g. if almost all the women belong to an extreme of the distribution. Hence the interest of ecological studies which compare the whole range of the distribution, for example those showing the international correlation between B.C. mortality rates and per capita fat consumption (Carrol et al., 1986). On the other hand, most of the commonly recognized risk factors, such as reproductive and dietary habits, have such a complex pattern of relationship with socio-cultural factors, that one cannot rule out the possibility that they are just a correlate of a still unrecognized environmental or life style determinant.

Most of these factors, whether actual causes of B.C. or just physiological or sociological correlates of the true causes, suggest that endogenous hormones, particularly those related to ovarian function, play an important role in altering the risk of the disease. The same hormones are essential for the normal development of the breast. It is not surprising therefore, that so many hypotheses have been developed in this field (Fig. 1).

The <u>adrenal androgens insufficiency</u> hypothesis postulates that 11-deoxy-17 ketosteroids, in particular DHEA, exert a protective effect. This theory arose in the late fifties, when the ratio of these hormones to 11-oxo--17-oxo steroids was shown to be predictive of B.C. response to endocrine surgery. It is based on some empirical evidence, mainly the results of the Guernsey Island prospective study (see further on) (Bulbrook et al., 1971; Spicer 1972) but has no physiopathological explanation. A few protective mechanisms have been postulated which are far from being proven: among them the competing effect of androstenediol, the 17-OH metabolite of DHEA, for estrogen receptors (Poortman et al., 1975) and the inhibiting effect of DHEA on glucose-6-phosphate-dehydrogenase activity, which may be essential for tumour metabolism (Cocco 1987) (Some association of B.C. with low 17 ketosteroids levels has been repeatedly found in premenopausal women (Zumoff 1982) but it has not been confirmed among postmenopausal women (De Waard and Banders-van Halewun 1974).

The anovulation-luteal inadequacy hypothesis postulates that P is protective by opposing the proliferative effects of EE on breast tissues, in analogy to what happens in the endometrium (Sherman and Korenman 1974; Mauvais-Jarvis et al., 1979). The theory is so appealing that several women are currently treated with progestinic drugs to prevent B.C.. Unfortunately there is no clear evidence of such an effect of P on the breast: in the luteal phase of the cycle, on the contrary, breast epithelium has a greater mitotic activity than in the follicular phase (Anderson et al., 1982). The finding of a hyperplastic proliferative endometrium in the second half of the cycle of most premenopausal women with B.C., as opposed to the usual secretory premenstrual pattern of normal women, strongly supported the theory (Grattarola 1964). One cannot exclude, however, that this pattern was a consequence, rather than a causal correlate, of B.C., possibly through the stressing conditions that accompany the discovery of the illness. The major difficulty of the theory is that case-control studies of pregnanediol in urine or of P in blood, yielded inconsistent results. P levels, however, may have such an important variation in normal women that gross misclassification is likely to occur in these studies (Filicori et al., 1984).

The same anatomical damage of the ovary postulated in the anovulation hypothesis, i.e. hyperplastic interstitial tissue with or without cysts, would be the cause of the increased androgenic activity leading to B.C. according to the ovarian androgens hypothesis (Grattarola 1972, 1973). Ovariectomy, in fact, reverses to normal both the increased androgenic excretion and the hyperplastic endometrial pattern observed in B.C. cases (Grattarola 1976).

According to this theory, high T levels coupled with low P levels in the second half of the cycle would determine the highest risk condition (Secreto et al., 1984).

Unfortunately the controversy between the sustainers of the protective effect of adrenal androgens and, respectively, the deleterious effect of ovarian androgens, lasted for twenty years without producing any study in which both androgenic families were contemporarily evaluated. All those who looked at serum or urinary T, within a case-control design, found higher levels among cases (Secreto et al., 1984; Hill et al., 1985; Adami et al., 1975; McFadyen et al., 1976; Fan et al., 1985; Malarkey et al., 1977). A study found no difference in the mean plasmatic T level of cases and controls, and was published as negative (Wang et al., 1966); however, it can be considered positive if distributions instead of means are considered (or if extreme values are excluded). These studies show fairly high RRs for women with high T levels of the order of 6 constrasting women above and under the 75th percentile. A small prospective study, however, has not confirmed the association (see further on) (Wysowski et al., 1987).

According to the E3 ratio (E3/(E1+E2)) hypothesis, E3 would have protective biological effects that are opposite to those of E1 and E2 (Lemon et al., 1966). High urinary E3 ratios are characteristic of pregnancy and this hypothesis dominated the epidemiological research since MacMahon and Cole produced evidence of the protective role of an early pregnancy (MacMahon et al., 1970). The theory was corroborated by several observations of high ratios among low risk populations, which decrease after migration into high risk countries (Trichopoulos et al., 1984). The assumption of an antiestrogenic action of E3 was later found to be wrong (Zumoff 1981). In fact the theory could not be confirmed by a fairly large case-control study which, on the contrary, found a moderately elevated B.C. risk in women with a high urinary level of both E3 and the other estrogens (Cole et al., 1978; MacMahon et al., 1983). Furthermore, most case-control studies failed to show any consistent association of B.C. with either urinary or blood levels of E2 or total estrogens (Zumoff 1981).

Despite this widespread inconsistency of epidemiological results, the total estrogen hypothesis still remains the most cherished theory of many researchers. The theory is supported by the efficacy of antiestrogenic therapy in some B.C. patients, by the preventive effect of ovariectomy (which, however, also modifies androgens) and by the changing pattern of B.C. incidence following natural menopause, but there is certainly no consensus that the levels of estrogens are elevated in either present or in future B.C. patients (Wysowski et al., 1987).

The unconventional estrogens hypotheses arose following the consideration that E1, E2 and E3 account for only half of the circulating estrogens. Catechol estrogens and methoxyderivatives are the main representatives of this group (Dao 1979). The metabolic pathways of E1 lead to 16 alpha-hydroxyestrone and E3 or, alternatively, hydroxylation at position two, to the catechol estrogens which are much less estrogenic than E3. The issue is of relevance to B.C. etiology because a number of environmental factors have been shown to affect the metabolism shifting the pathway towards catechol estrogens (e.g. tobacco smoking) or towards E3 (e.g. fat diet and obesity) (Bradlow et al., 1986). The theory is indirectly supported by the observations that obese postmenopausal women have an increased risk of B.C. and that cigarette smoking women may have a slightly lower risk (IARC 1985).

The estrogen windows hypothesis was a brilliant tentative to overcome the difficulties of both the estrogenic and progestinic theories. It postulates that breast tissue is responsive to environmental carcinogenic stimuli only in the two periods in which estrogens are not "opposed" by P because of a high frequency of anovulatory cycles: a few years after menarche and before menopause (Korenman 1980). The protection conferred by late menarche, early first pregnancy and early menopause, would depend on the shortening of these anovulatory periods. The observation that teenagers are more susceptible than older women to ionizing radiation supported the theory (Boice et al., 1979). Hiroshima girls who were under the age of ten, that is before menarche, at the time of the bombing, however, later proved to have been more susceptible too (Tokunaga et al., 1982). An alternative explanation of the susceptibility of young women, therefore, must be postulated. The observation that early menarche is associated with an earlier establishment of regular ovulatory cycles (Aptor and Vihko 1983) instead of a later one, pushed the estrogen window hypothesis out of fashion. Perimenarche conditions and events, however, remain a very promising field of hypotheses for future studies on B.C. etiology. There are indications, in fact, that physical exercise (Frisch et al., 1985) and low calorie intake (de Waard et al., 1986) at or around menarche may have a protective effect.

The difficulties of the estrogen windows theory, together with the results of a case-control study showing a higher risk of B.C. in young women taking estroprogestinic oral contraceptives (Pike et al., 1983), led to the formulation of a provocative progestinic hypothesis, according to which P would cause B.C. instead of preventing it (Henderson et al., 1985). This theory had the merit of shaking the fragile empirical and conceptual basis of previous theories, but was itself based on indirect evidence only.

Meanwhile, a new star was arising, the free E2 hypothesis, according to which, only the non SHBG bound fraction of estrogens, i.e. the fraction allegedly available to the target organs, is relevant to B.C. etiology (Siiteri et al., 1981).

This theory aroused much enthusiasm and a number of small case control studies, usually badly designed, were rapidly produced (Siiteri et al., 1981; Moore et al., 1982; Reed et al., 1983; Langley et al., 1985; Ota et al., 1986; Pearce et al., 1987), which with a few exceptions (Bruning et al., 1985; Jones et al., 1985), showed high free E2 and/or low SHBG levels among cases. Eventually a unifying theory emerged that, apparently, could accommodate observations both on T and the inconsistent findings on estrogens; high T levels, in fact, decrease SHBG production and, as T has a much greater affinity for SHBG than E2, may displace the latter from the protein, thereby increasing its free fraction. Preliminary results from the Guernsey Island prospective study (see further on) seemed to corroborate this theory (Bulbrook et al., 1984; Moore et al., 1986b).

The issue, however, is far from being understood: There are also negative studies and, most of all, the physiologic basis of the theory is being challenged by the same authors who proposed it (Siiteri 1987). Actually, it is not known if SHBG helps or contrasts the peripheral utilization of sex hormones.

The prevailing opinion, today, seems to be, that the total amounts of hormones in the urine or in the peripheral blood are only marginally related to B.C. risk (Moore et al., 1986a) and other theories are being considered, focusing on the concentration of hormones within breast tissues, or, alternatively, on the susceptibility of breast epithelium to hormones. They are mainly based on the observation that the intramammary concentration of a few hormones, mainly estrogens, is much higher (up to 20 times) than blood concentration (Vermeulen 1986). The capability of breast tissue to utilize plasmatic hormones, such as E1 sulphate, is also actively investigated (Santen 1986).

Waiting for a better definition of these new hypotheses, which today do not seem easily feasible with an epidemiological design, it would not be wise to reject all past results as confused and obscure; instead, the reasons for inconsistency should be attentively scrutinized.

Most studies did not pay much attention to the selection of cases and controls, with respect to the major determinant of B.C. risk and of hormonal levels. The size of the studies was usually small and many researchers did not consider the issue of statistical power. Only a few studies controlled for circadian and circamenstrual variation. The possible confounding effect of one class of hormones, when looking at another class of hormones, has almost never been taken into account. Individual variability over time has never been thoroughly studied: nobody knows what the predictive value is of a single or a few hormonal determinations to identify women with a given hormonal unbalance. Also, the dramatic effect of misclassification has rarely been considered: a 75% sensitivity, for instance, to detect women in the upper quartile of the distribution, would cause an underestimation of a RR of 50 to 7.5, or, respectively, a RR of 10 to 4.4 (contrasting women above and under the 75th percentile). In a recent study (Berrino et al., 1988), TS, DHT, adione and TU were measured twice in the same woman, two years apart. The correlation was good for TS ($r = 0.73$), DHT ($r = 0.80$) and adione ($r = 0.70$), but was much poorer for urinary androgens.

Most hormonal theories were fairly satisfactory in providing reasonable explanations of the main physiological correlates of B.C. risk. The protection conferred by pregnancy, for instance, apparently fitted with the E3 ratio hypothesis (E3 levels are very high in pregnancy), with luteal inadequacy (which would be a cause of both B.C. and low parity), with the ovarian androgens hypothesis (anovulating ovaries produce more androgen), with estrogen window (an early pregnancy would produce an early closure of the first window), with the free hormones hypothesis (nulliparous women have lower SHBG levels than multiparous women) and with the prolactin hypothesis (after the huge levels reached in pregnancy, the prolactin levels of parous women remain persistently lower than among nullipaorus women). It would appear to be an extremely debatable topic, but apparently the biological plausibility does not help to choose the correct theory.

PROSPECTIVE STUDIES

A major draw-back of case-control studies on hormones and B.C. is that one can never rule out the possibility that the illness itself, or the stress associated with the diagnosis, is responsible for the observed differences between cases and controls.

Follow-up studies, or case-control studies within a prospective cohort, where biological samples are collected before diagnosis of B.C., in principle, should avoid this bias. They have the further advantage of allowing the comparison of incident cases with their source population, instead of with a surrogate control group.

Unfortunately only a few prospective observations are available on hormones and B.C..

In 1961 a prospective study was undertaken in the Island of Guernsey (Bulbrook et al., 1971) where urine specimens were collected from 5 000 women.

When a case of breast cancer was subsequently diagnosed, the patient's specimen was retreived from storage together with a various number of matched controls. Assays for androsterone, etiocholanolone and DHEA were then carried out. Ten years from the start of the study 27 women had developed B.C., and it was shown that their excretion of androsterone and etiocholanolone was significantly lower than that of controls (Bulbrook et al., 1971). A later publication allows the computation of relative risks for dichotomous categories of etiocholanolone, specific for two classes of age (up to 44, 45 and over) and three of parity (nulliparous, first pregnancy before 25 years of age, and first pregnancy at 25 years or more) (Spicer 1972). As etiocholanolone excretion decreases with age whilst B.C. incidence increases, a residual confounding by age cannot be excluded. However, the study shows that nulliparous women and women with a late first pregnancy who excrete less etiocholanolone (roughly the lower tertile) have a three-fold risk of B.C. with respect to women who excrete more (RR = 3.2, 95% C.I. 1.5-6.6). The effect is greater among young women than among older women. No effect can be observed among women who had an early pregnancy (RR = 0.7, 95% C.I. 0.1-3.9). Overall, the age and pregnancy adjusted RR is 2.4 (95% C.I. 1.2 4.6). These are probably the most valid results that have been produced up to now by epidemiological studies on hormones and B.C. Unfortunately the association does not seem strong enough to explain the broad international differences of B.C. incidence (see Fig. 4).

The Guernsey Island study was later expanded to collect blood and store serum samples at $-20°C$. About 5 000 women have been enrolled. The first 13 women who developed B.C. had a higher proportion of their blood E2 in the free and albumin-bound fractions, compared with controls (Bulbrook et al., 1984). This was accompanied by diminished SHBG concentration (Moore et al., 1986b). Unfortunately, as was later clarified (Bulbrook 1987), the association was confined to B.C. cases diagnosed at the time of enrollment, or occurred in the following four years: but in the following years no further association was present.

A prospective study carried out in Washington County, Maryland, U.S.A. was recently published on 13 000 women, 73 of which developed B.C. during a follow-up of 7 years (Wysowski et al., 1987). The analysis was confined to 17 premenopausal and 39 menopausal women. No significant difference was found for E1, E2, E3, and P, which however, were slightly lower among cases, nor for adione and T. The study was not designed to study B.C., time at which blood was taken was not mentioned, the analysis was carried out only to compare mean hormone values, sera were examined in two different laboratories, 21 cases were not examined to spare sera, but the criteria with which they have been chosen were not specified. Notwithstanding these defects, the study suggests that serum levels may be of little importance and that more sophisticated prospective studies should be carried out.

Further prospective studies are in progress in Utrecht, The Netherlands (DOM project, de Waard et al., 1974); New York, U.S.A. (Shore et al., 1983) and Varese, Italy (ORDET study, Berrino et al., 1988).

CONCLUSIONS

The relationship between sex steroid hormones and B.C. is a very complex one, which refuses to fit in with any etiological hypothesis without leaving unexplained or contrary facts.

Historically the rise of new theories follows the development of analytical techniques: for instance that seems to have been the case for adrenal androgens, E3 ratio, unconventional estrogens and free E2. In the last 35 years we have witnessed a continuous technical progress, from the early colorimetric methods of measuring estrogens in urine, to gas-chromatography, to radioimmunoassays, which made the measuring of blood concentration possible, to the identification of biological active fractions, and to mass spectrography. Today the availability of techniques for measuring hormonal concentration and steroid metabolism within the tumour itself, or within normal breast tissue, together wth the unsatisfactory results of three decades of conventional hormonal assays, prompts the development of new hypotheses focusing on tissue concentration and on tissue sensitivity to circulating hormones; rather than on urinary and blood levels. Such hypotheses are more difficult to challenge from an epidemiological point of view. Indicators of hormone peripheral activity, such as sebum production, hirsutism, body fat distribution, height, height when seated, may provide some hint, but specific indicators of tissue susceptibility, which are not easy to obtain from normal women, are clearly needed. Studies of hormonal composition

(Petrakis et al., 1987) of nipple aspirates or of breast cyst fluid (Rossner et al., 1985) are in progress; however, they too may be just an indirect indicator of breast metabolism and susceptibility. Individual response to normal or abnormal hormonal levels, on the other hand, may be genetically determined, and the development of DNA restriction fragment length polymorphism techniques will provide further clues to the interpretation of the relationship of hormonal milieu and B.C. Future epidemiological studies should include the collection of DNA samples to be analysed for genetic polymorphism when the relevant probes will be available.

Most of all, it would not have much sense, in future studies, to look at androgens only and ignore estrogens, and vice versa. All the relevant hormonal fractions should be determined, paying attention to storage conditions and to the standardization and quality control of laboratories. It would not have much sense either to repeat small studies without knowing to which extent cases and controls belong to the same population base, or without collecting relevant information on the commonly recognized correlates of B.C. and of hormonal levels, or without taking into account the timing of biological samples within the day or the month.

Most studies so far carried out have ignored the question as to whether or not a single analytical determination, (or determinations within a single day or month) has any value in correctly classifying a woman on her usual or relevant hormonal pattern. We have only little idea as to whether, and to what extent, negative or insignificant results may depend on random misclassification (Muti et al., 1988). Studies on intraindividual variability, therefore, should be encouraged.

Hormonal levels may vary according to environmental or psychological conditions such as diet, smoking, stress and unrelated ilness. A number of studies have tried to choose controls as normal as possible, but what about the normality of cases?

It is clear that a prospective design, based, for example, on a biological bank, would consent to sample controls from the source population of cases. Information on potentially confounding factors should be available, which, however, is not often the case in large prospective studies. A prospective design would also avoid the major obstacle in interpreting hormonal case-control studies, i.e. the question as to whether hormonal alterations precede B.C. or are caused by the tumour itself, or by some tumour associated condition, such as diagnostic or therapeutic stress.

In prospective studies, however, data on hormonal profile would be scattered over a period of many years before the diagnosis of B.C.. Again this would be informative only if the predictive value of a single or a few determinants are high (relative to the biochemical defect which should be detected).

The size of prospective studies is necessarily limited by the huge costs of establishing and maintaining a biological bank for many years. International cooperation to plan large studies is certainly preferable to the proliferation of small studies lacking essential information for the full interpretation of the results.

REFERENCES

Adami, H.O., Johansson, E.D.B., Vegelius, J. and Victor, A. (1979) Serum concentrations of estrone, androstenedione, testosterone and sex-hormone-binding-globulin in postmenopausal women. Upsalla J. Med. Sci., 84, 259-274

Anderson, T.J., Ferguson, D.J.P. and Raab, G.M. (1982) Cell turnover in the 'resting' human breast: influence of parity, contraceptive pill, age and laterality. Br. J. Cancer, 46, 376-382

Apter, D. and Vihko, R. (1983) Early menarche, a risk factor for breast cancer, indicates early onset of ovulatory cycles. J. Clin. Endocrinol. Metab., 57, 82-87

Berrino, F., Pisani, P., Muti, P., Crosignani, P. and Panico, S. (1988) ORDET: Prospective study of hormones and diet in the etiology of breast cancer. Synthesis of the project. This Volume.

Boice, Jr., J.D., Land, C.E., Shore, R.E., Norman, J.E. and Kokunaga, M. (1979) Risk of breast cancer following low-dose radiation exposure. Radiology, 131, 589-597

Bondy, P.K. (1985) Disorders of the adrenal cortex. In: J.D. Wilson and D.W. Foster. Williams Text Book of Endocrinology. pp. 816-890, W.B. Saunders Co., Philadelphia, U.S.A.

Bradlow, H.L., Hershcopt, R.E. and Fishman, J.F. (1986) Oestradiol 16-alpha-hydroxylase: a risk marker for breast cancer. Cancer Surveys, 5, 573-583

Bradlow, H.L. (1987) Steroid protein interactions: The first 50 years. International Congress on Steroid Protein Interactions. Sept. 29th - Oct. 1st, 1987, Turin, Italy.

Breslow, N.E. and Day, N.E. (1980) Statistical methods in cancer research, Vol. 1. The analysis of case-control studies. IARC Scientific Publications No. 32, Lyon, France.

Bruning, P.F., Bonfrer, J.M.G. and Hart, A.A.M. (1985) Non protein-bound estradiol, sex-hormone-binding-globulin. Br. J. Cancer, 51, 479-484

Bulbrook, R.D., Hayward J.L. and Spicer, C.C. (1971) Relation between urinary androgen and corticosteroid excretion and subsequent breast cancer. Lancet, ii, 395-597

Bulbrook, R.D., Moore, J.W., Wang, D.Y. and Clark, G.M.G. (1984) Oestrogens and the aetiology and clinical course of breast cancer. In: M. Borzsonyi, K. Lapis, N.E. Day and H. Yamasaki (eds). Models, Mechanisms and Etiology of Tumour Promotion. IARC Scientific Publications No. 56, Lyon, France.

Bulbrook, R.D. (1987) International congress on steroid protein interaction. 29th Sept. - 1st Oct. 1987, Turin, Italy. Personal Communication.

Carroll, K.K., Braden, L.M., Bell, J.A. and Kalamegham, R. (1986) Fat and cancer. Cancer, 58, 181801825

Cocco, P. (1987) Does G6PD deficiency protect against cancer? A critical review. J. Epidemiol. Commun. Health, 41, 89-93

Cole, P., Cramer, D., Yen, S., Paffenberger, R., MacMahon, B and Brown, J. (178) Estrogen profiles of premenopausal women with breast cancer. Cancer Res., 38, 745-748

Dao, T.J. (1979) Metabolism of estrogens in breast cancer. Biochimica et Biophysica Acta, 560, 397-426

De Waard, F., Collette, H.J. and Rombach, J.J. (1986) Het Domproject voor de vroege opsporing van borst kanker to Utrecht. Utrecht, 1986.

De Waard, F. and Banders-van Halewun, E.A. (1974) A prospective study in general practice on breast cancer risk in postmenopausal women. Int. J. Cancer, 14, 153-160

Fan, C., Shu-shi, W., Qing-tai, D., Li-ying, X., Wan-ying, L., Wen-xiu, Y., Zhen-guo, W. and Feng-yi, Y. (1985) A study on plasma sex hormone levels in patients with breast cancer. Chinese Med. J., 98, 507-510

Filicori, M., Butler, J.P. and Crowley, W.F. (1984) Neuroendocrine regulation of the corpus luteum in the human. Evidence for pusatile progesterone secretion. J. Clin. Invest., 73, 1638-1647

Frisch, R., Wyshak, G., Albright, N.L., Albright, T.E., Schiff, I., Jones, K.P., Witschi, J., Shiang, E., Koff, E. and Marguglio, M. (1985) Lower prevalence of breast cancer and cancers of the reproductive system among former college athletes compared to non-athletes. Br. J. Cancer, 52, 885-891

Fritz, D.A. and Speroff, L. (1982) The endocrinology of menstrual cycle: the interaction of folliculogenesis and neuroendocrine mechanisms. Fertility and Sterility, 38, 509-520

Grattarola, R. (1964) The premenstrual endometrial pattern of women with breast cancer: a study of preogestational activity. Cancer, 17, 1119-1122

Grattarola, R. (1972) Androgenic cause of breast carcinoma and endometrial hyperplasia. Cancer Cytology, 12, 15-18

Grattarola, R. (1973) Androgens in breast cancer. 1. Atypical endometrial hyperplasia and breast cancer in married premenopausal women. Am. J. Obstet. Gynecol., 116, 423-428

Grattarola, R. (1976) Ovariectomy alone or in combination with dexamethasone in patients with advanced breast cancer and high levels of testosterone excretion. J. Nat. Cancer Inst., 56, 11

Henderson, B.E., Ross, R.K., Judd, H.L., Krailo, M.D. and Pike, M.C. (1985) Do regular ovalatory cycles increase breast cancer risk? Cancer, 56, 1206-1208

Hill, P., Garbaczewski, L. and Kasumi, F. (1985) Plasma testosterone and breast cancer. Eur. J. Cancer Clin. Oncol., Vol. 21, 1265-1266

IARC (1985) IARC Monographs on the Evaluation of the Carcinogenic Risk of Chemicals to Humans, Vol. 38, Tobacco smoking, IARC, Lyon, France

Jones, L.A., Ota, D.M., Jackson, G.A., Kemp, K. and Bauman, D.H. (1985) % non-protein bound and % albumin bound estradiol as a possible biomarker for breast cancer. 8th Annual San Antonio breast cancer symposium. Breast Cancer Res. Treat., 6, 180 (Abstract)

Kelsey, J.L. and Hildreth, G.N. (1983) Breast and gynecologic cancer epidemiology. CRC Press, Boca Raton, Florida, U.S.A.

Kirschner, M.A. (1979) The role of hormones in the development of human breast cancer. In: W.L. McGuire, (ed), Breast Cancer, Advances in Research and Treatment, Plenum Medical Book Co., New York, Vol. 3, 199-226

Korenman, S.G. (1980) Oestrogen window hypothesis of the aetiology of breast cancer. Lancet, i, 700-701

Langley, M.S., Hammond, G.L., Bardsley, A., Sellwood, R.A. and Anderson, D.C. (1985) Serum steroid binding proteins and the bioavailability of estradiol in relation to breast diseases. J. natl. Cancer Inst., 75 823-829

Lemon, H.M., Wotiz, H.H., Parsons, L. and Mozden, P.J. (1966) Reduced estriol excretion in patients with breast cancer prior to endocrine therapy. J. American Med. Assoc., 196, 1128-1136

MacMahon, B., Lin, T.M., Lowe, C.R., Miua, A.P., Ravnihar, B., Siber, E.J., Valoras, V.G. and Yuasa, S. (1970) Age at first birth and breast cancer risk. Bull, WHO., 43 209-221

MacMahon, B., Cole P., Brown, J.B., Paffenbarger, R., Trichopoulos, D. and Yen, S. (1983) Urine estrogens, frequency of ovulation, and breast cancer risk: case-control study in premenopausal women. J. natl. Cancer Inst., 70. 247-250

Malarkey, W.B., Schroeder, L.L., Stevens, V.C., James, A.G. and Lanese, R.R. (1977) Twenty-four hour preoperative endocrine profiles in women with benign and malignant breast disease. Cancer Res., 37, 4655-4659

Mauvais-Jarvis, P., Sitruk-Ware, L.R., Kutenn, F. and Sterkers, N. (1979) Luteal phase insufficiency: a common pathophysiological factor in benign and malignant breast disease. In: R.D. Bulbrook and J.D. Taylor (eds). Commentaries on Research in Breast Disease. Alan, R. Liss, New York, pp. 25-29

McFadyen, I.M., Prescott, R.J., Groom, G.V., Forrest, A.P.M., Golder, M.P., Fahmy, D.R. and Friffiths, K. (1976) Circulating hormone concentrations in women with breast cancer. Lancet, i, 100-1101

Miller, A.B. (1987) Breast cancer epidemiology, etiology and prevention. In: J. Harris, S. Hellman, C.I. Henderson and D. Kinne (eds). Breast Diseases. Philadephia, Lippincott Co. pp. 87-102

Moore, J.W., Clark, G.M.G., Bulbrook, R.D., Hayward, J.L., Murai, J.T., Hammond, G.L. and Siiteri, P.K. (1982) Serum concentrations of total and non-proteine-bound oestradiol in patients with breast cancer and in normal controls. Int. J. Cancer, 29, 17-21

Moore, J.W., Thomas, B.S. and Wang, D.Y. (1986a) Endocrine status of breast cancer. Cancer Surveys, 5, 536-559

Moor, J.W., Clark, G.M.G., Hoare, S.A., Millis, R.R., Hayward, J.L., Quinlan, M.K., Wang, D.Y. and Bulbrook, R.D. (1986b) Binding of oestradiol to blood proteins and the aetiology of breast cancer. Int. J. Cancer. 38 625-630

Muti, P., Pisani, P., Crosignani, P., Michell, A., Panico, S., Secreto, G. and Berrino, F. (1988) ORDET - Prospective study on hormones, diet and breast cancer: feasibility study and long term quality control. Steroids, accepted for publication.

Ota, D.M., Jones, L.A., Jackson, G.L., Jackson, P.M., Kemp, K. and Bauman, D. (1986) Obesity, non-protein-bound estradiol in the sera of breast cancer patients. Cancer, 57, 558-562

Pearce, S., Dowsett, M., Mackinna, J.A. and Feffcats, S.L. (1987) Non-proteine-bound oestradiol and testosterone in breast cancer patients and matched controls. 176th Meeting of the Society for Endocrinology. J. Endocrinol., 115 (Supplement): Abstract 72

Petrakis, N.L., Ernster, V., King, M. (1982) Breast. In: D. Schottenfield and J.F. Fraumeni (eds). Cancer epidemiology and prevention. W.B. Saunders Co., Philadelphia, U.S.A., pp. 855-870

Petrakis, N.L., Wrensch, M.R., Ernster, V.L., Miike, R., Rurai, J., Simberg, N. and Siiteri, P.K. (1987) Influence of Pregnancy and lactation on serum and breast fluid estrogen levels: implications for breast cancer risk. Int. J. Cancer, 40, 587-591

Pike, M.C., Henderson, B.E., Krailo, M.D. and Duke, A. (1983) Breast cancer in young women and use of oral contraceptives: possible modifying effects of formulation and age at use. Lancet, ii, 926-930

Poortman, J., Prenen, A.C., Schwarz, F. and Thijssen, J.H.H. (1975) Interaction of delta 5-androstene-3 beta, 17- beta-diol with estradiol and dihydrotestosterone receptors in human myometrium and mammary cancer tissue. J. Clin. Endocrinol. Metab., 40, 373-379

Reed, M.J., Cheng, R.W., Noel, C.T., Dudley, H.A.F. and James, V.H.T. (1983) Plasma levels of estrone, estrone sulphate and estradiol and th percentage of unbound estradiol in post-menopausal women with and without breast cancer. Cancer Res., 43, 3940-3943

Rosner W., Khan, S.M., Breed, C.N., Fleisher, M. and Bradlow, H.L. (1985) Plasma steroid-binding proteins in the cysts of gross cystic disease of the breast. J. Clin. Endocrinol. Metab., 61, 200-203

Santen, R.J. (1986) Determinants of tissue oestradiol levels in hyman breast cancer. Cancer Surveys, 5, 597-615

Secreto, G., Toniolo, P., Berrino, F., Recchione, C., Di Pietro, S., Fariselli G. and Decarli, A. (1984) Increased androgenic activity and breast cancer risk in premenopausal women. Cancer Res., 44, 5902-5905

Sherman, B.M. and Korenman, S.G. (1974) Inadequate corpus luteum function: a pathophysiological interpretation of human breast cancer epidemiology. Cancer, 33, 1306-1312

Shore, R.E., Pasternack, B.S., Bulbrook, R.D., Moseson, M., Kwa, H.G., Wang, D.Y., Moore, J.W. and Strax, P. (1983) Endocrine and environmental factors in breast cancer: the case for prospective studies. In: R.D. Bulbrook and D.J. Taylor (eds). <u>Commentaries on Research in Breast Disease</u>, Alan R. Liss Inc., New York, N.Y., U.S.A., <u>3</u>, 2-31

Siiteri, P.K., Hammond G.L. and Nisker, J.A. (1981) Increased availability of serum estrogens in breast cancer: a new hypothesis. In: M.C. Pike, P.K. Siiteri and C.W. Welsch (eds). <u>Hormones and Breast Cancer</u>, Banbury Report 8, Cold Spring Harbor Laboratory, Cold Spring Harbor, N.Y. U.S.A.

Siiteri, P.K. (1987) Estrogen transport and action in humans. International Congress on Steroid Protein Interaction. 29th Sept. 1987, Turin, Italy. Personal Communication.

Spicer, C.C. (1972) Androagens and age at first birth in relation to risk of breast cancer. In: R.Doll and I. Vodopija (eds). <u>Host Environment Interactions in the Etiology of Cancer in Man</u>. IARC Scientific Publications No. 7, Fogarty International Center Proceedings No. 18, 159-162, IARC, Lyon, France

Tokunaga, M., Land, C.E., Yamamoto, T., Asano, M., Tokuoka, S., Ezaki, H. and Hishimori, I. (1982) Breast cancer in Japanese A-bomb survivors. <u>Lancet</u>, <u>ii</u>, 924

Trichopoulos, D., Yen, S., Brown, J., Cole, P. and MacMahon, B. (1984) The effect of westernization on urine estrogens, frequency of ovulation, and breast cancer risk. <u>Cancer</u>, <u>53</u>, 187-192

Vermeulen, A. (1986) Human mammary cancer as a site of sex steroid metabolism. <u>Cancer Surveys</u>, <u>5</u>, 585-616

Wang, D.Y., Hayward, J.L. and Bulbrook, R.D. (1966) Testosterone levels in the plama of normal women and patients with benign breast disease or with breast cancer. <u>Eur. J. Cancer</u>, <u>2</u>, 373-376

Waterhouse, J., Muir, C., Shanmugaratnman, K. and Powell, J. (1982) Cancer incidence in five continents. Volume IV. IARC Scientific Publications No. 42. IARC, Lyon, France.

Wysowski, D.K., Comstock, G.W., Helsing, K.J. and Lau, H.L. (1987) Sex hormone levels in serum in relation to the development of breast cancer. <u>Am. J. Epidemiol.</u>, <u>125</u>, 791-799

Yen, S.C. and Faffe, R.B. (1986) Reproductive Endocrinology. W.B. Saunders Co., Philadelphia, U.S.A.

Zumoff, B. (1981) The role of endogenous estrogen excess in human breast cancer (Review). <u>Anticancer Res.</u>, <u>1</u>, 39-40

Zumoff, B. (1982) Hormone profiles and the epidemiology of breast cancer. In: B.A. Stoll (ed). <u>Endocrine Relationships in Breast Cancer</u>, pp. 3-47, William Heinemann Med. Books, London

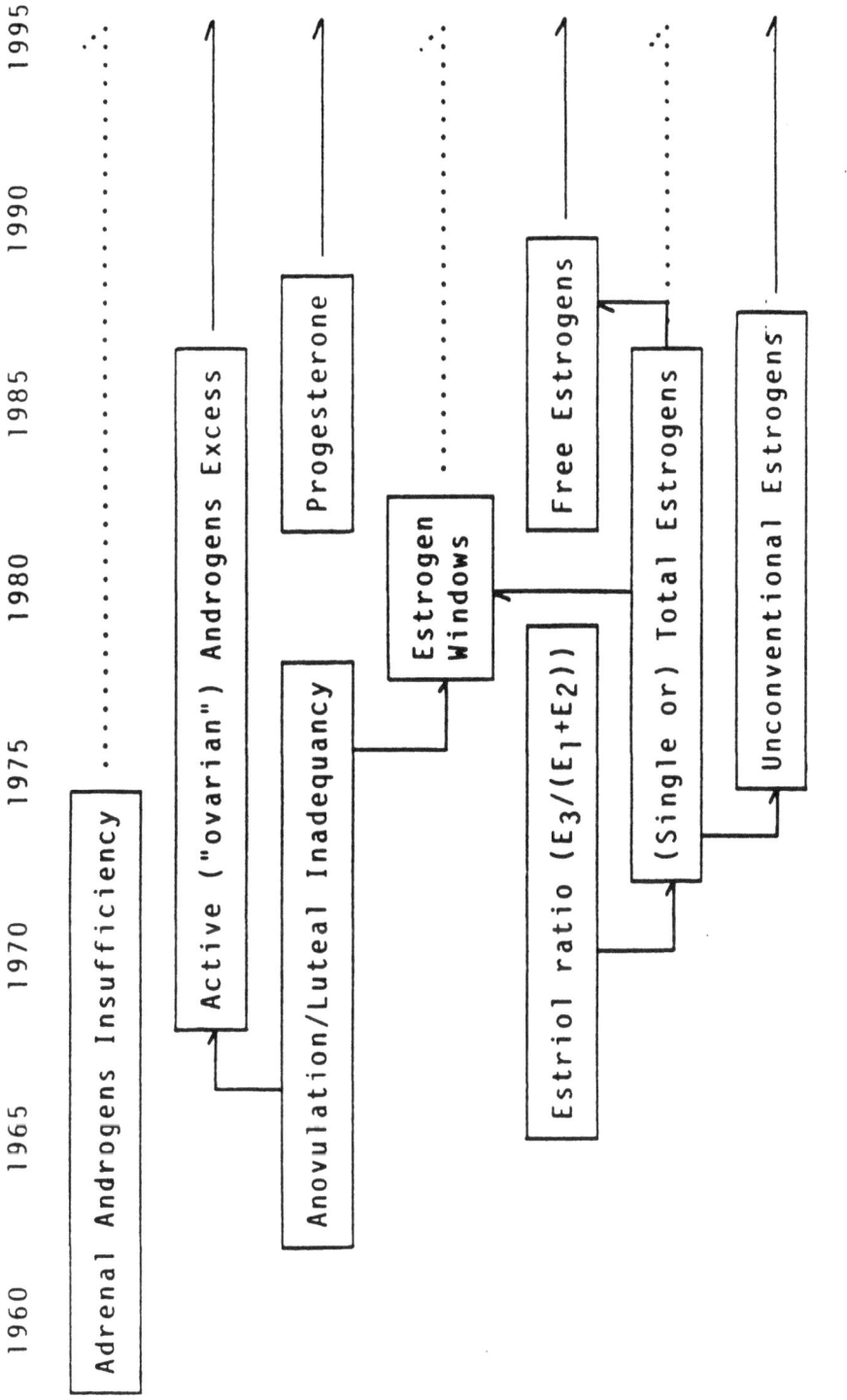

Fig. 1 - Sex steroid hormones and breast cancer: history of hormonal theories.

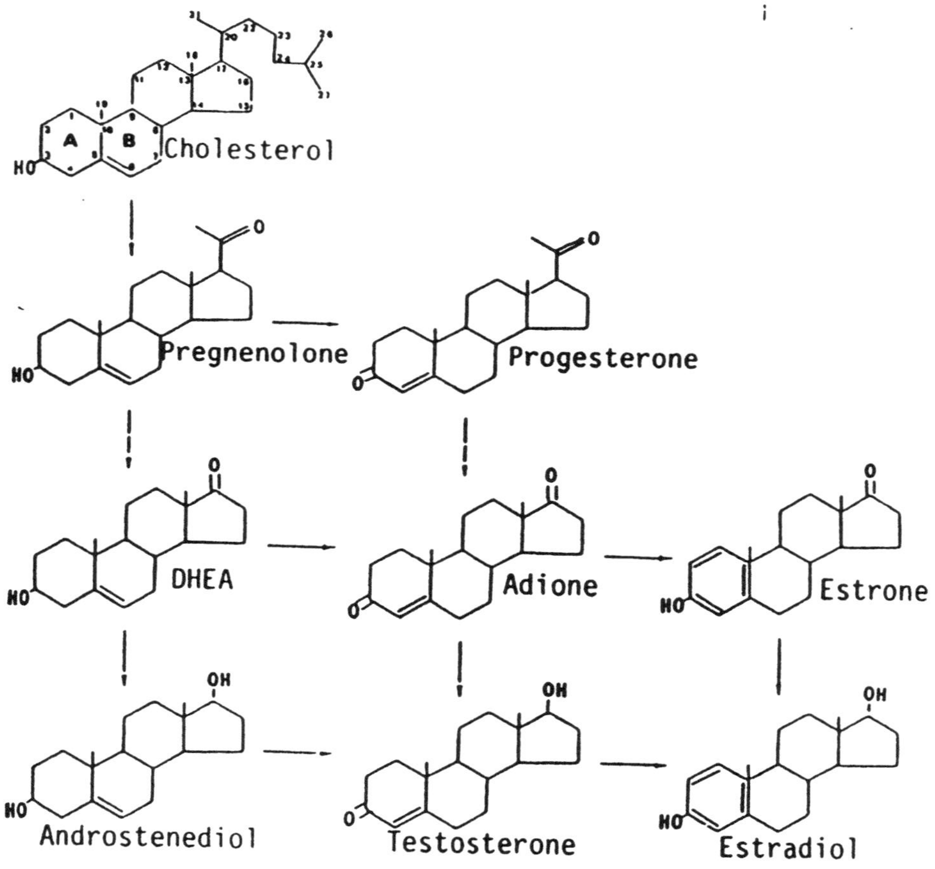

Fig. 2 - Biosynthesis of sex steroid hormones.

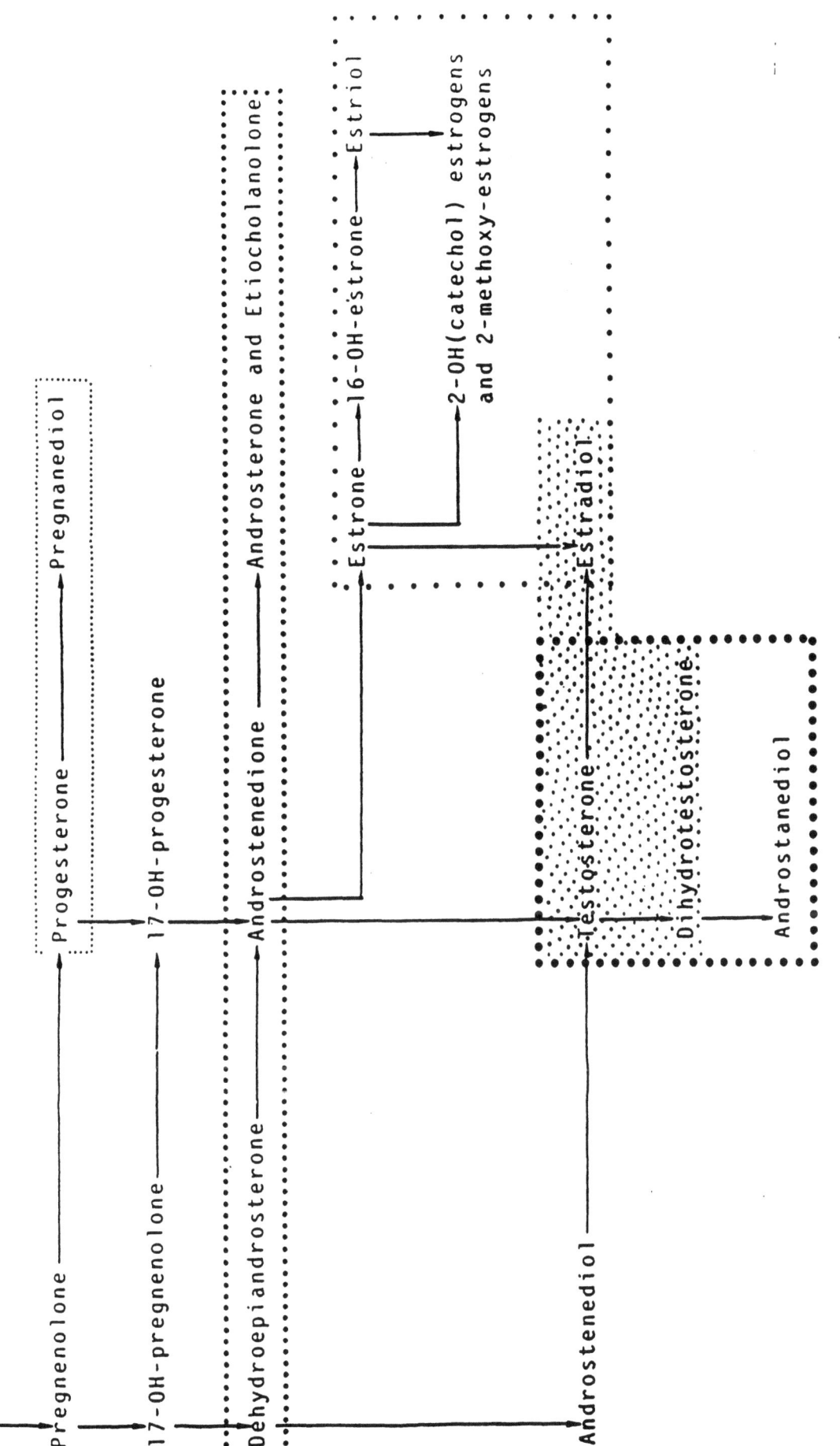

Figure 3. Main biosynthetic pathways of sex steroid hormones. Dotted lines indicate the hormonal families to which the hypotheses listed in Fig. 1 refer i.e. the progestogens area, the "adrenal" 17 keto androgens area, the major androgens area, and the estrogens area. The dotted area indicates the Sex Hormon Binding Globulin bound hormones.

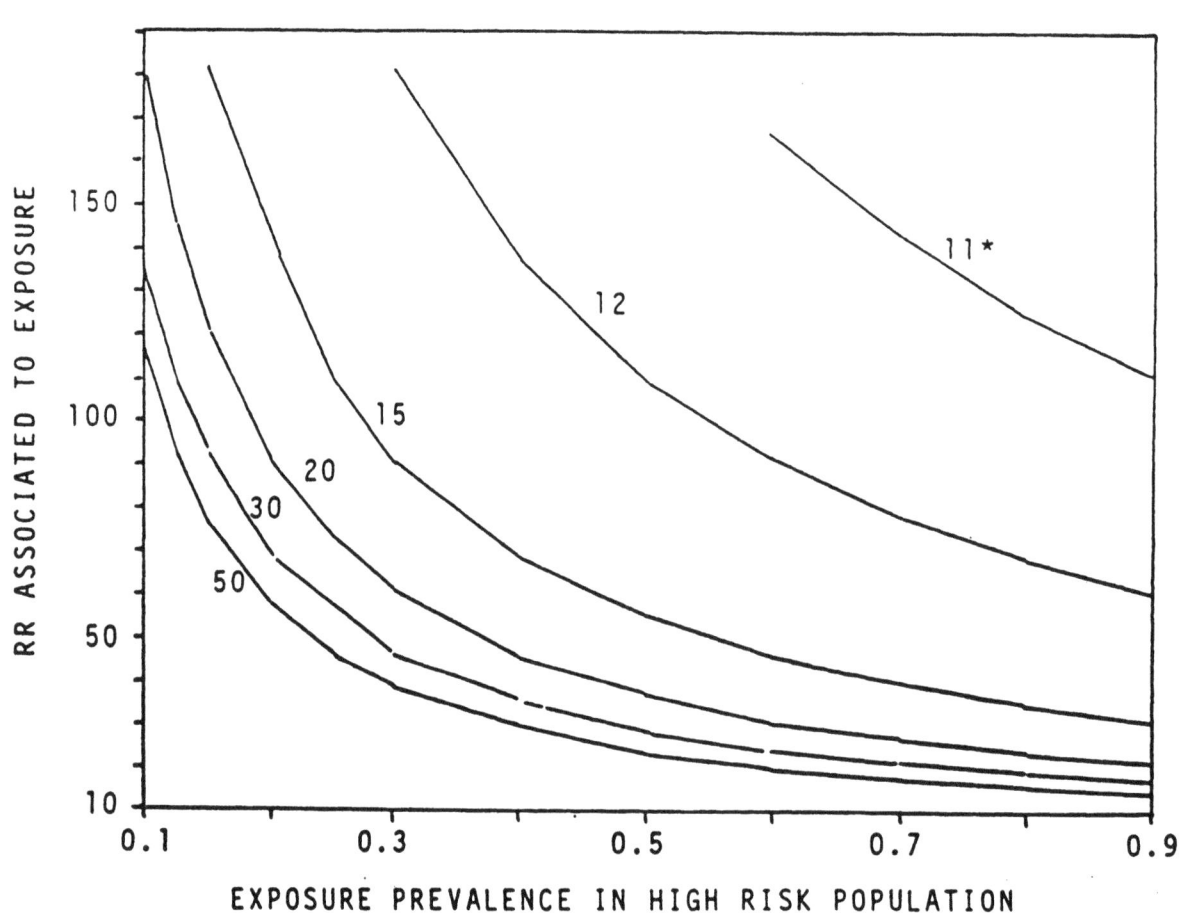

FIG. 4 - RR NECESSARY TO EXPLAIN A TENFOLD INCIDENCE RATIO IN TWO POPULATIONS GIVEN DIFFERENT EXPOSURE PREVALENCES

*(Exp.Prev. in high risk pop.)/(Exp.Prev. in low risk pop.)

EXOGENOUS SEX HORMONES AND CANCER:
RECENT FINDINGS ON SEX HORMONE BINDING GLOBULIN,
RISK FACTORS FOR BREAST CANCER, AND ORAL CONTRACEPTIVES

T.J.A. Key

Imperial Cancer Research Fund, Cancer Epidemiology Unit, Gibson Building, Radcliffe Informary, Oxford OX2 6HE, UK

Dr F. Berrino has introduced sex hormone binding globulin (SHBG) as one component of an etiological hypothesis linking endogenous sex hormones and breast cancer. The possible importance of SHBG was first proposed by Siiteri et al. (1981): they suggested that a low concentration of SHBG may increase the risk of developing breast cancer by increasing the proportion of oestradiol which is free to reach the breast epithelial cells. We have measured the SHBG concentration in serum samples from the 5000 women in the Imperial Cancer Research Fund's prospective study of breast cancer in the Island of Guernsey (see Moore et al., 1986), and looked for relationships between SHBG and other known or possible risk factors for breast cancer.

We initially restricted our analysis to the 1221 subjects who had never used oral contraceptives (OCs) or hormone replacement therapy (HRT). In this subset of subjects we confirmed previous observations of a strong inverse relationship between SHBG and body mass index (BMI) and of an increase in SHBG during the luteal phase of the menstrual cycle.

We found that SHBG is higher (+12%) in parous than in nulliparous premenopausal women (adjusting for BMI, day of cycle and age at menarche, one-sided $p = 0.004$), but that the lower SHBG of the nulliparous premenopausal women is confined to those who are unmarried. In postmenopausal women the mean SHBG of all nulliparous women does not differ from that of parous women, but again the unmarried nulliparous postmenopausal women have a lower SHBG than the married nulliparous postmenopausal women (adjusting for BMI and years since menopause, one-sided $p = 0.001$). Bernstein et al. (1985) also reported that SHBG is higher in parous than in nulliparous young women; most of the nulliparous women in their study were unmarried. The possibility that SHBG is related to marital status rather than to parity is unexpected and requires confirmation.

We found that in premenopausal women SHBG is higher in women who had a late menarche than in those who had an early menarche (test for linear trend using actual age at menarche and adjusting for BMI, parity, marital status and day of cycle, one-sided $p = 0.058$) and is higher in smokers than in non-smokers (adjusting for BMI, age at menarche, parity, marital status and day of cycle, one-sided $p = 0.051$). No significant differences in SHBG according to age at menarche or smoking habit were found in postmenopausal women.

After examining our data for women who had never used exogenous sex hormones, we then looked at the effects of current and past use of OCs and HRT on SHBG. We found, as expected, that SHBG is higher in current users of HRT and of oestrogen-containing OCs than in non-current users. SHBG is not affected by previous use of HRT, but women who have previously used OCs have a lower mean SHBG than never users as shown in Table 1 (premenopausal - adjusting for BMI, parity, marital status, age at menarche, age, and day of cycle, one-sided $p = 0.008$; postmenopausal - adjusting for BMI, parity, marital status, and years since menopause, one-sided $p = 0.036$). This long-term effect of OCs on SHBG does not vary with the number of years for which OCs were used or with the number of years since OCs were last used. There were no statistically significant differences according to the brand of OC used, but our results suggest that the long-term decrease in SHBG only follows use of OCs containing at least 50 micrograms of ethinyloestradiol or at least 100 micrograms of mestranol. Cole et al. (1978) reported another long-term effect of OCs: they found that urinary oestrogen excretion was much lower in women who had previously used OCs for more than 1.5 years than in never-users of OCs. These long-term effects of OCs on oestrogen metabolism must be considered when interpreting studies of the relationships between OCs and breast cancer.

REFERENCES

Bernstein, L., Pike, M.C., Ross, R.K., Judd, H.L., Brown, J.B. & Henderson, B.E. (1985) Estrogen and sex hormone-binding globulin levels in nulliparous and parous women. J. Natl. Cancer Inst., 74, 741-745

Cole, P., Cramer, D., Yen, S., Paffenbarger, R., MacMahon, B. & Brown, J. (1978) Estrogen profiles of premenopausal women with breast cancer. Cancer Res., 38, 745-748

Moore, J.W., Clark, G.M.G., Hoare, S.A., Millis, R.R., Hayward, J.L., Quinlan, M.K., Wang, D.Y. & Bulbrook, R.D. (1986) Binding of oestradiol to blood proteins and etiology of breast cancer. Int. J. Cancer, 38, 625-630

Siiteri, P.K., Hammond, G.L. & Nisker, J.A. (1981) Increased availability of serum estrogens in breast cancer: a new hypothesis. In: Pike, M.C., Siiteri, P.K. & Welsch, C.W., eds, Hormones and Breast Cancer (Banbury Report 8), Cold Spring Harbor Laboratory, New York

Table 1. Relationship between sex hormone binding globulin (SHBG) and previous use of oral contraceptives (OCs)

OC use	Premenopausal		Postmenopausal	
	SHBG[a]	No. of subjects	SHBG[b]	No. of subjects
Never	68.2	616	58.8	779
Previous	65.1	1244	54.5	115
	66.1	1860	58.2	894

[a] Mean value (nmol/l), adjusted for body mass index, parity, marital status, age at menarche, age, and day of cycle.

[b] Mean value (nmol/l), adjusted for body mass index, parity, marital status, and years since menopause.

EXOGENOUS DETERMINANTS OF PREGNANCY OESTROGENS
AND THEIR RELEVANCE TO CANCER ETIOLOGY. A STUDY IN GREECE

D. Trichopoulos[1] & E. Petridou[2]

[1]Department of Hygiene and Epidemiology, University of Athens Medical School, Goudi, Athens 115 27, Greece

[2]Division of Maternal and Child Health, PIKPA Organization

INTRODUCTION

In 1986 the Department of Hygiene and Epidemiology of the University of Athens and the Division of Maternal and Child health of the PIKPA National Welfare Organization of Greece started a prospective study of the role of diet and tobacco smoking as possible determinants of pregnancy oestrogens and of the height and weight of the newborn. The authors of this communication are the coordinators of the project, in collaboration with Dr K. Panayotopoulou of PIKPA, Dr E. Spanos of Biomedicine Ltd., and Associate Professor A. Antzaklis of the Alexandra Maternity Teaching Hospital. Professor B. MacMahon of the Harvard School of Public Health has kindly agreed to act as consultant to the research team on various matters concerning the whole project.

BACKGROUND

The scientific justification of the study is based on a series of empirical and possibly causal relationships, described below and summarized in Fig. 1.

Endogenous oestrogens are probably involved in the etiology of female breast cancer

The theory that endogenous oestrogens play a crucial role in the etiology of human breast cancer is based on indirect and direct evidence. The indirect evidence derives from experimental work in laboratory animals (Loeb, 1940; Bittner, 1955; Dao, 1981), from medical experience and clinical investigations (reviewed by MacMahon and Cole, 1972), from epidemiological studies of exogenous oestrogens (Hoover et al., 1976; Jick et al., 1980; Ross et al., 1980), and from epidemiological studies linking biological indicators of endogenous oestrogen stimulus (e.g. age at menarche, age and type of menopause) to breast cancer risk (Kelsey, 1979). The indirect evidence is in itself overwhelming, but there are questions concerning its relevance to the ovarian etiology of human breast cancer. Thus, species differences must be accounted for before any extrapolation from experimental animals is attempted; clinical studies on the oestrogen responsiveness of established tumours may not be relevant to cancer initiation and promotion; exogenous oestrogens may be different in terms of bio-availability and biological activity from endogenous oestrogens; and physiological processes like pregnancy, menarche and menopause may be indicators of other endocrine and metabolic parameters besides oestrogens.

The direct evidence is based on actual measurements of oestrogens in human subjects, is usually of an epidemiological nature, and is inherently relevant to the human disease. There are three types of studies of this nature: population (risk) correlations, case-control, and cohort studies. Several oestrogen correlation studies have been undertaken (Dickinson et al., 1974; MacMahon et al., 1974; Henderson et al., 1975; Kelsey, 1979) and most of them have lent support to the idea that oestrogens are somehow involved in the etiology of human breast cancer - although none of them was sensitive enough to discriminate between alternative oestrogen-oriented etiological hypotheses (e.g. importance of total oestrogens, or oestrone alone, or of the oestriol ratio). However, the demonstrative power of population correlations under the best of conditions is rather limited.

Several case-control studies have compared urine or plasma levels of oestrogens between women with breast cancer and control women (about ten studies). These studies have been reviewed by Kirschner (1977), Cole et al. (1978) and Zumoff (1981), who felt that on the whole the results were inconclusive. However, if these results are weighted according to the corresponding study size, appropriateness of control group, attention to timing in specimen collection and quality of laboratory procedures, the overall pattern of findings is considerably more supportive of the idea that endogenous oestrogens are important in human breast carcinogenesis. Thus England et al. (1974) found higher serum oestrogens in premenopausal and postmenopausal women with breast cancer, whereas Morreal et al. (1979) found elevated urine oestrogens in postmenopausal women with breast cancer. Moore et al. (1982) noted that serum oestradiol is significantly raised in postmenopausal women whereas non-protein-bound oestradiol (Siiteri et al., 1981) is increased in both pre- and postmenopausal women (there is evidence that total urine oestrogens correlate better with the "biologically available" non-bound oestrogen (Armstrong et al., 1981)). Finally, MacMahon et al. (1982) found a clear and significant discrimination between breast cancer patients and unaffected women when actual oestrogen levels (rather than oestriol ratios or pregnanediol values) were considered in the data analysis.

Diet appears to be one of the most important exogenous determinants of breast cancer incidence, but the specific nutrients or food groups involved have not been established

Cancer of the breast is among the most common cancers worldwide (Parkin et al., 1984). Studies in migrants indicate that little, if any, of the international variation may be accounted for by genetic factors (Trichopoulos et al., 1984). Several exogenous risk factors have been identified but they appear collectively inadequate to explain a major part of the variability of the disease (Kelsey & Hildreth, 1983). Diet is now considered by most investigators to be perhaps the most important exogenous determinant of breast cancer incidence because: (i) breast cancer incidence correlates strongly with fat consumption and other nutrient intakes in international series (Armstrong & Doll, 1975; Doll & Peto, 1981); (ii) weight and other diet-related factors have been found to correlate with breast cancer risk in several analytical epidemiology studies (de Waard, 1981); (iii) adipose tissue appears to be involved in the endocrinology that may affect breast cancer genesis and progression (de Waard, 1981; de Waard, 1982; Santen, 1982); and (iv) in several animal models, diet and particularly fat appears to be an important factor in mammary carcinogenesis (Committee on Diet, Nutrition and Cancer, 1982). However, the results of analytical epidemiology studies focusing on diet have been much less conclusive, and specific nutrients or food groups with a clear etiological role have not been identified with certainty.

Diet may affect endogenous oestrogen levels and/or production rats, but no clear pattern of association has emerged

Since both oestrogens and diet appear to be major factors in the etiology of breast cancer (as well as of other cancers including endometrial cancer) it seems reasonable to consider whether diet may exercise its postulated effect, at least in part, through modulation of endogenous oestrogen levels and/or production rates. Several studies have been undertaken in order to explore this important issue but the results have been inconclusive (Armstrong et al., 1981; Goldin et al., 1981; Goldin et al., 1982; Adlercreutz et al., 1986). This should not be unexpected, even if diet were a strong determinant of oestrogen levels; in addition to the well known problems involved in assessing dietary intakes there are major difficulties in measuring the minute amounts of oestrogens in blood specimens. Furthermore, these specimens must be carefully "timed" in order to account for the "cyclical" variation of oestrogens, in step with the frequently irregular menstrual pattern.

In the menstruating woman tobacco smoking reduces oestrogens; this may explain the association of smoking with several oestrogen-related diseases (e.g. endometrial cancer) and conditions (e.g. age at menopause, osteoporosis)

MacMahon et al. (1982) found that tobacco smoking substantially reduces the levels of urinary oestrogens, mainly during the luteal phase of the menstrual cycle. Michnovicz et al. (1986) reported the anti-oestrogenic effect of tobacco smoking during both the follicular and the luteal phase of the menstrual cycle, and attributed it to increased 2-hydroxylation of oestradiol (Fig. 2). Among postmenopausal women smoking was found by Jensen et al. (1985) to increase degradation of exogenous oestrogens, resulting in correspondingly lower plasma oestrogen levels. These findings provide a ready explanation for the reported protective effect of tobacco smoking against endometrial cancer, as well as for the well known association between tobacco smoking and osteoporosis and early menopause (Baron, 1984; Weiss, 1985).

The association between tobacco smoking and breast cancer has been examined in a number of studies, but the results have been equivocal (MacMahon et al., 1982; Baron, 1984; Weiss, 1985; Berkowitz et al., 1985; Hiatt & Fireman, 1986). Before interpreting these findings as contradictory to the hypothesis implicating endogenous oestrogens in the etiology of breast cancer, several issues must be addressed:
(1) Among men, smoking has been associated with hyper- rather than with hypo-oestrogenaemia (Lindholm et al., 1982; Klaiber et al., 1984) and among postmenopausal women Trichopoulos et al. (1987) found no negative association between tobacco smoking and urinary oestrogens (which, in these women, are mostly of extraovarian origin). Therefore, if endogenous oestrogens are indeed involved in the etiology of breast cancer, it will be reasonable to expect a slight negative association between smoking and breast cancer risk only, or mainly, among premenopausal women.
(2) Among women with breast cancer, tobacco smoking is strongly related to oestrogen receptor status (Daniell, 1980). Therefore, receptor status must be taken into account, as an interacting factor, in any study exploring the role of smoking in the etiology of breast cancer.
(3) The postulated smoking effect is small, and confounding due to reproductive and dietary factors (including alcohol) may be substantial. Therefore, large and specifically designed studies may be needed in order to demonstrate the smoking effect - if one does actually exist.

Diet is an important determinant of birth height and weight; and maternal cigarette smoking has been found to be strongly associated with decreased birth height and weight

Obese women tend to have large babies and, among normal women, a baby's birth weight is related to the woman's weight gain during pregnancy. Furthermore, encouraging lean women to achieve an appropriate weight gain reduces the proportion of low birth weight babies, whereas dietary restriction during pregnancy can reduce the birth weight of the babies (Drife, 1986).

Maternal cigarette smoking has been found repeatedly to be strongly associated with decreased birth height and weight (Persson et al., 1978; Rush & Cassano, 1983). The association appears to be independent of social class and is not confounded by other factors that could theoretically cause certain women both to smoke and to produce smaller babies (Rush & Cassano, 1983; Wainwright, 1983). Several mechanisms have been postulated in order to explain the association between maternal smoking on the one hand and birth height and weight on the other (Rush & Cassano, 1983); most of them focus on nutritional disturbances, but placental structural changes and smoking effects on the embryo have also been invoked. It should be noted, however, that there is little empirical evidence to support any of the above stated pathogenetic mechanisms.

THE HYPOTHESIS AND THE PROJECT

The hypothesis investigated in this project is based on the following postulates (Trichopoulos, 1986):
(1) During pregnancy, oestrogens, which are established growth factors in many biological systems, are important determinants of foetal growth and, therefore important determinants of birth height and weight.
(2) Factors such as diet and tobacco smoking, which appear to affect oestrogen levels and/or production rates in the menstruating woman, are also important determinants of oestrogens during pregnancy.

The hypothesis is biologically plausible and may explain several epidemiological observations, including the following: (i) Active smoking (which can reduce oestrogens in the menstruating woman (MacMahon et al., 1982)) is also negatively related to birth height and weight (Persson et al., 1978; Rush & Cassano, 1983; Wainwright, 1983). (ii) The disproportionally strong effect of passive maternal smoking on birth weight (Martin & Bracken, 1986; Rubin et al., 1986; Trichopoulos, 1986) may be accounted for by methodological factors, but it may also be due to the fact that during pregnancy most oestrogens are metabolized through the 16-alpha-hydroxylation pathway (leading to the production of abundant oestriol (Fig. 2), and thus allow substantial marginal potential for the postulated tobacco-induced 2-hydroxylation (and subsequent production of the much less oestrogenic 2-hydroxyoestrone and 2-methoxyoestrone) (Speroff et al., 1983; Michnovicz et al., 1986). (iii) There appears to be a population (risk) correlation between oestrogen levels in menstruating women and median values of birth height and weight.

The present project, the pilot stage of which is now approaching completion, has the basic structure of a cohort study. Extensive demographic, socio-economic and medical data are collected, dietary (semi-quantitative food frequency) questionnaires are completed, and information about active and passive smoking is obtained from pregnant women at an advanced stage of their pregnancy. Oestrogen fractions, total oestrogens, human placental lactogen and other biochemical variables are measured in the blood of these women during the 26th and 31st week of their pregnancy. Finally, several data concerning the newborn are registered, including height and weight.

If the oestrogens of menstruating women and pregnancy oestrogens have indeed some common determinants, the design used in the present project will offer several methodological advantages including a relatively recent reference period for dietary assessment, an inherently short latent period, and a relatively high (and therefore easier to measure) levels of oestrogens. The pregnant woman may not be a perfect model for the non-pregnant woman (with respect to oestrogen determinants), but the proposed approach avoids the problems introduced by inter-species differences when extrapolation from laboratory animal experimentation is attempted.

If the outlined hypothesis is even partially true, the present project and, in more general terms, the proposed study model may allow the identification of some determinants of a number of oestrogen-related diseases or conditions (early menopause, osteoporosis, endometrial cancer, breast cancer, other cancers, etc.). Even if pregnancy oestrogens have few common determinants with the oestrogens of the menstruating woman the project may provide some useful information concerning factors affecting pregnancy oestrogens and/or the newborn's height and weight.

ACKNOWLEDGEMENT

This study is supported by a grant from the Ministry of Youth, Greece.

REFERENCES

Aldercreutz, H., Fotsis, T., Bannwart, C., Hamalainen, E., Bloigu, S. & Ollus, A. (1986) Urinary estrogen profile determination in young Finnish vegetarian and omnivorous women. J. Steroid Biochem., 24, 289-296

Armstrong, B.K., Brown, J.B., Clarke, H.T. et al. (1981) Diet and reproductive hormones: a study of vegeterian and nonvegetarian postmenopausal women. J. natl. Cancer Inst., 67, 761-767

Armstrong, B. & Doll, R. (1975) Environmental factors and cancer incidence and mortality in different countries with special reference to dietary practices. Int. J. Cancer, 15, 617-631

Baron, J.A. (1984) Smoking and estrogen-related diseases. Am. J. Epidemiol., 119, 9-22

Berkowitz, G., Canny, P., Vivolsi, V., Merino, M., O'Connor, T. & Kelsey, J. (1985) Cigarette smoking and benign breast disease. J. Epidemiol. Commun. Hlth, 39, 308-313

Bittner, J.J. (1955) Experimental aspects of mammary cancer in mice. In: Lewison, E.L., ed, Breast Cancer and its Diagnosis and Treatment, Baltimore, Williams & Wilkins, pp. 75-102

Cole, P., Cramer, D., Yen, S., Paffenbarger, R., MacMahon, B. & Brown, J. (1978) Estrogen profiles of premenopausal women with breast cancer. Cancer Res., 38, 745-748

Committee on Diet, Nutrition and Cancer, National Research Council (1982) *Diet, Nutrition and Cancer*, Washington, D.C., National Academy Press

Daniell, H.W. (1980) Estrogen receptors, breast cancer and smoking. *N. Engl. J. Med.*, *302*, 1478

Dao, T.L. (1981) *The role of ovarian steroid hormones in mammary carcinogenesis*. In: Pike, M.C., Siiteri, P.K. & Welsch, C.W., eds, *Hormones and Breast Cancer (Banbury Report 8)*, New York, Cold Spring Harbor Laboratory, pp. 281-295

De Waard, F. (1981) *Body size and breast cancer risk*. In: Pike, M.C., Siiteri, P.K. & Welsch, C.W., eds, *Hormones and Breast Cancer (Banbury Report 8)*, New York, Cold Spring Harbor Laboratory, pp. 21-26

De Waard, F. (1982) Nutritional etiology of breast cancer: where are we now and where are we going? *Nutr. Cancer*, *4*, 85-89

Dickinson, L.E., MacMahon, B., Cole, P. & Brown, J.B. (1974) Estrogen profiles of Oriental and Caucasian women in Hawaii. *N. Engl. J. Med.*, *291*, 1211-1213

Doll, R. & Peto, R. (1981) The causes of cancer: quantitative estimates of avoidable risks of cancer in the United States today. *J. natl. Cancer Inst.*, *66*, 1191-1308

Drife, J.O (1986) Weight gain in pregnancy: eating for two or just getting fat? *Br. Med. J.*, *293*, 903-904

England, P.C., Skinner, L.G., Cottrell, K.M. & Sellwood, R.A. (1974) Serum oestradiol-17 beta in women with benign and malignant breast disease. *Brit. J. Cancer*, *30*, 571-576

Goldin, B.R., Adlercreutz, H., Dwyer, J.T., Swenson, L., Warram, J.H. & Gorbach, S.L. (1981) Effect of diet on excretion of estrogen in pre- and postmenopausal women. *Cancer Res.*, *41*, 3771-3773

Goldin, B.R., Adlercreutz, H., Gorbach, S.L., Warram, J.H., Dwyer, J.T., Swenson, L. & Woods, M.N. (1982) Estrogen excretion patterns and plasma levels in vegetarians and omnivorous women. *N. Engl. J. Med.*, *307*, 1542-1547

Henderson, B.E. Gerkins, V., Rosario, I., Casagrande, J. & Pike, M.C. (1975) Elevated serum levels of estrogen and prolactin in daughters of patients with breast cancer. *N. Engl. J. Med.*, *293*, 790-795

Hiatt, R. & Fireman, B. (1986) Smoking, menopause and breast cancer. *J. natl. Cancer Inst.*, *76*, 833-838

Hoover, R., Gray, L.A., Cole, P. & MacMahon, B. (1976) Menopausal estrogens and breast cancer. *N. Engl. J. Med.*, *295*, 401-405

Jensen, J., Christiansen, C. & Rodbro, P. (1985) Cigarette smoking, serum estrogens, and bone loss during hormone-replacement therapy early after menopause. *N. Engl. J. Med.*, *313*, 973-975

Jick, H., Walker, A.M., Watkins, R.N. et al. (1980) Replacement estrogens and breast cancer. *Am. J. Epidemiol.*, *112*, 586-594

Kelsey, J.L. (1979) A review of the epidemiology of human breast cancer. Epidemiol. Rev., 1, 74-109

Kelsey, J.L. & Hildreth, N.G. (1983) Breast and Gynecologic Cancer Epidemiology, Boca Raton, FL, CRC Press Inc.

Kirschner, M.A. (1977) The role of hormones in the etiology of human breast cancer. Cancer, 39, 2716-2726

Klaiber, E., Broverman, D. & Dalen, J. (1984) Serum estradiol levels in male cigarette smokers. Am. J. Med., 77, 858-862

Lindholm, J., Winkel, P., Brodthagen, U. & Gyntelberg, F. (1982) Coronary risk factors and plasma sex hormones. Am. J. Med., 73, 648-651

Loeb, L. (1940) The significance of hormones in the origin of cancer. J. natl. Cancer Inst., 1, 169-195

MacMahon, B. & Cole, P. (1972) The ovarian etiology of human breast cancer. Rec. Res. Cancer Res., 39, 185-192

MacMahon, B., Cole, P., Brown, J.B. et al. (1974) Urine oestrogen profiles of Asian and North American women. Int. J. Cancer, 14, 161-167

MacMahon, B., Cole, P., Brown, J., Paffenbarger, R., Trichopoulos, D. & Yen, S. (1982) Urine estrogens, frequency of ovulation and breast cancer risk. J. natl. Cancer Inst., 70, 247-250

MacMahon, B., Trichopoulos, D., Cole, P. & Brown, J. (1982) Cigarette smoking and urinary estrogens. N. Engl. J. Med., 307, 1062-1065

Martin, T.R. & Bracken, M.B. (1986) Association of low birth weight with passive smoke exposure in pregnancy. Am. J. Epidemiol., 124, 633-642

Michnovicz, J., Hershcopf, R., Naganuma, H., Bradlow, H. & Fishman, J. (1986) Increased 2-hydroxylation of estradiol as a possible mechanism for the anti-estrogenic effect of cigarette smoking. N. Engl. J. Med., 315, 1305-1309

Moore, J.W., Clark, G.M.G., Bulbrook, R.D. et al. (1982) Serum concentrations of total and non-protein-bound oestradiol in patients with breast cancer and in normal controls. Int. J. Cancer, 29, 17-21

Morreal, C.E., Dao, T.L., Nemoto, T. & Lonergan, P.A. (1979) Urinary excretion of estrone, estradiol, and estriol in postmenopausal women with primary breast cancer. J. natl. Cancer Inst., 63, 1171-1174

Parkin, D.M., Stjernwsard, J. & Muir, C.S. (1984) Estimates of the worldwide frequency of twelve major cancer. Bull. WHO, 62, 163-182

Persson, P.H., Grennert, L., Gennser, G. & Kullander, S. (1978) A study of smoking and pregnancy with special reference to fetal growth. Acta Obstet. Gynecol. Scand. Suppl., 78, 33-39

Ross, R.K., Paganini-Hill, A., Gerkins, V.R. et al. (1980) A case-control study of menopausal estrogen therapy and breast cancer. J. Am. Med. Assoc., 243, 1635-1639

Rubin, D.H., Krasilnikoff, P.A., Leventhal, J.M., Weile, B. & Berget, A. (1986) Effect of passive smoking on birth weight. Lancet, ii, 415-417

Rush, D. & Cassano, P. (1983) Relationship of cigarette smoking and social class to birth weight and perinatal mortality among all births in Britain. J. Epidemiol. Commun. Hlth, 37, 249-255

Santen, R.J. (1982) Overall experience with aminoglutethimide in the management of advanced breast carcinoma. I: Mechanisms of action. In: Elsdon-Dew, R.W., Jackson, I.M. & Birwood, G.E.B., eds, Aminoglutethimide: An Alternative Endocrine Therapy for Breast Carcinoma, International Congress and Symposium Series No. 53, London, The Royal Society of Medicine, pp. 3-7

Siiteri, P.K., Hammond, G.L. & Nisker, J.A. (1981) Increased availability of serum estrogens in breast cancer: A new hypothesis. In: Pike, M.C., Siiteri, P.K. & Welsch, C.W., eds, Hormones and Breast Cancer (Banbury Report 8), New York, Cold Spring Harbor Laboratory, pp. 87-101

Speroff, L., Glass, R.H. & Kase, N.E. (1983) Clinical Gynecologic Endocrinology, 3rd Edition, Baltimore, Williams & Wilkins

Trichopoulos, D. (1986) Passive smoking, birth weight and oestrogens. Lancet, ii, 743

Trichopoulos, D., Yen, S., Brown, J., Cole, P. & MacMahon, B. (1984) The effect of Westernization on urine estrogens, frequency of ovulation, and breast cancer risk (A study of ethnic Chinese in the Orient and the U.S.A.). Cancer, 53, 187-192

Trichopoulos, D., MacMahon, B. & Brown, J. (1987) Urine estrogens and breast cancer risk factors among postmenopausal women (submitted for publication).

Wainwright, R.L. (1983) Change in observed birth weight associated with maternal cigarette smoking. Am. J. Epidemiol., 117, 675-688

Weiss, N.S. (1985) Can not smoking be hazardous to your health? N. Engl. J. Med., 313, 632-633

Zumoff, B. (1981) The role of endogenous estrogen excess in human breast cancer (review). Anticancer Res., 1, 39-44

Figure 1. Some established and postulated links between diet, tobacco smoking, endogenous oestrogens and oestrogen-related diseases or conditions

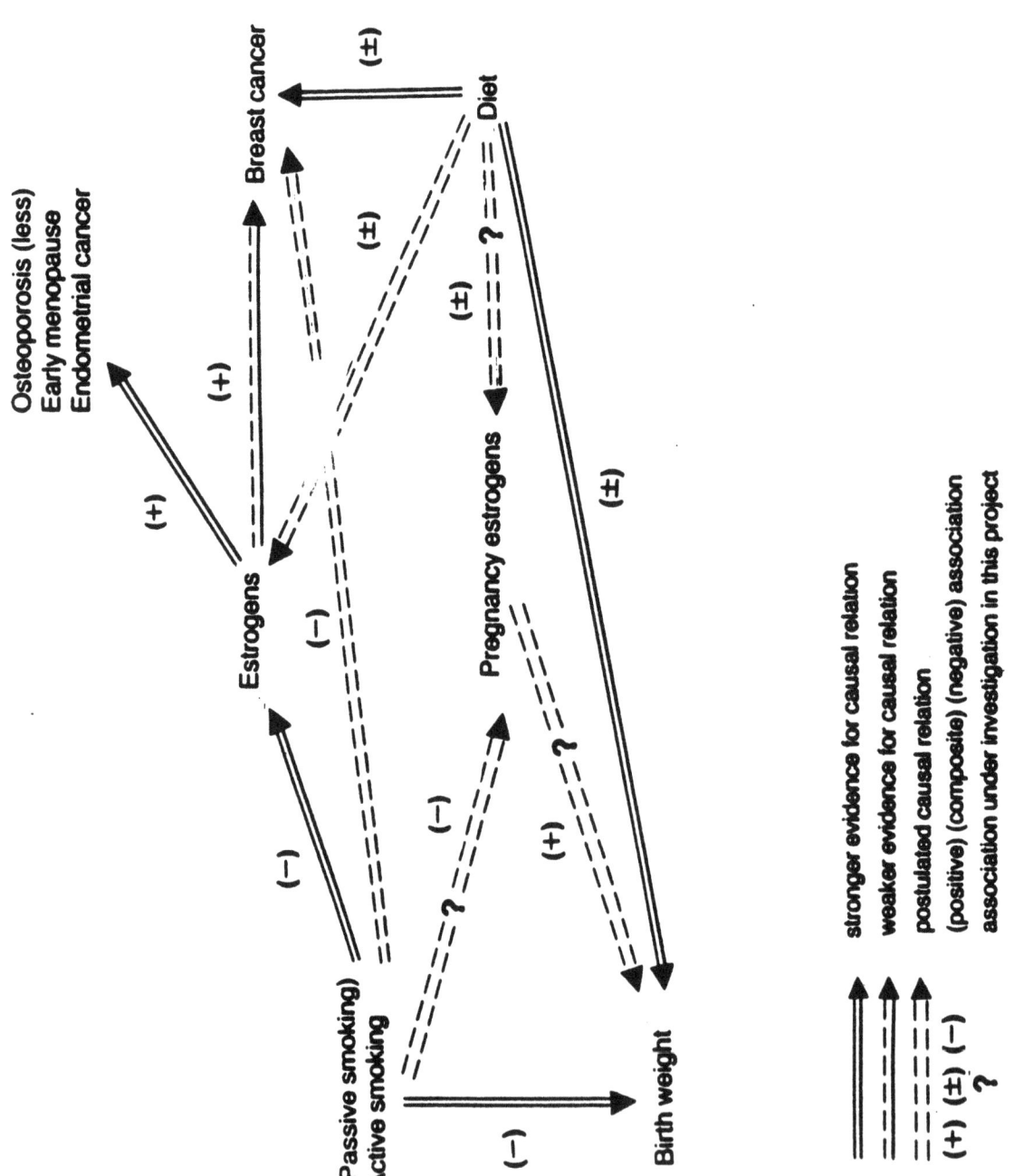

Figure 2. Oxidative transformations of oestradiol in women (Michnovicz et al., 1986)

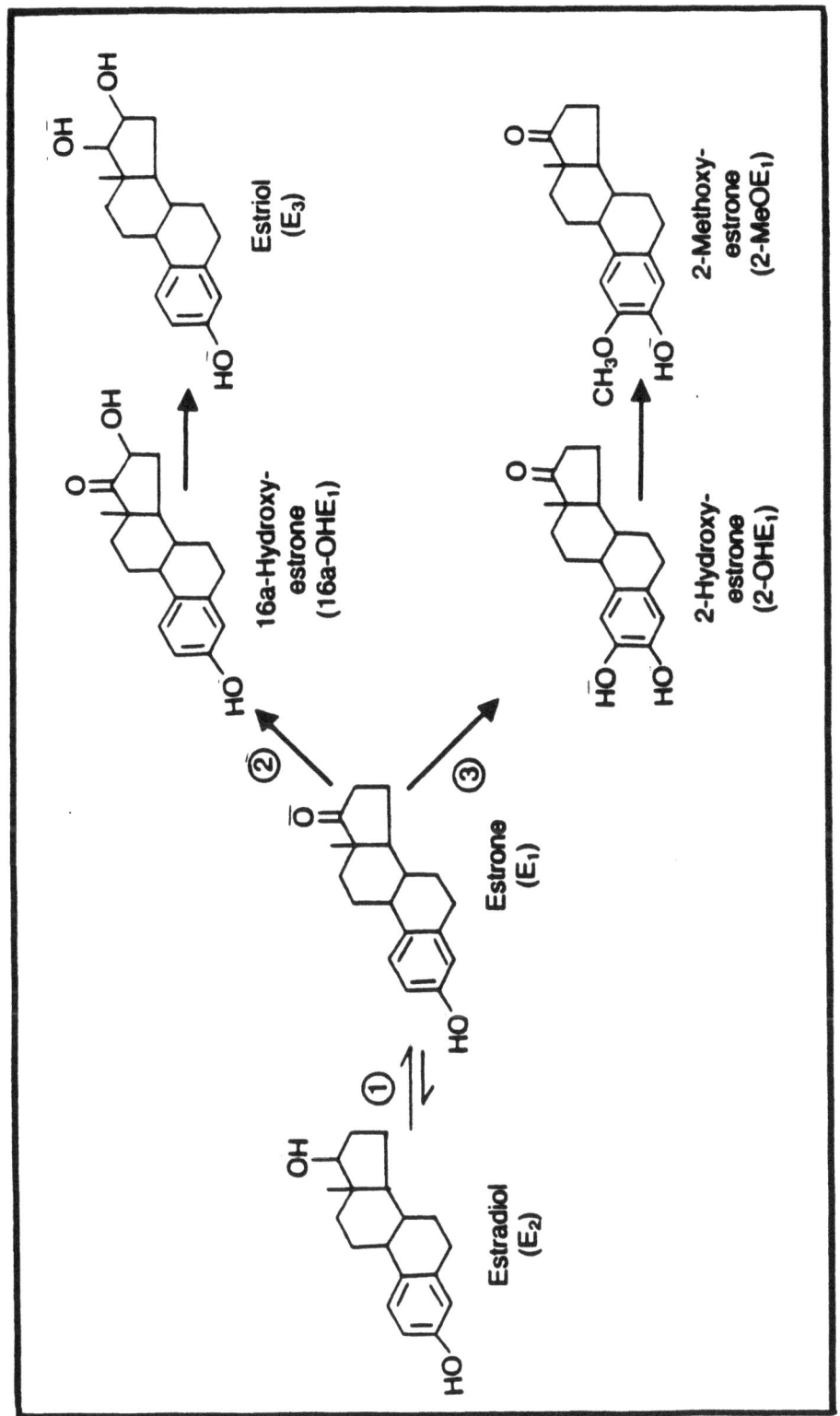

HORMONES AND CANCER
MULTIPLE PRIMARY CANCERS OF THE FEMALE REPRODUCTIVE ORGANS

Marianne Ewertz

Danish Cancer Registry, 66 Landskronagade, 2100 Copenhagen Ø, Denmark

For over a hundred years it has been recognized that the tendency to multiple primary cancers in some individuals provides a clue to the understanding of cancer etiology. If individuals with one cancer show an increased risk of a second primary cancer at a different site, it may be inferred that the two cancers have etiological factors in common or that agents used in the treatment of the first cancer are carcinogenic.

Cohort studies conducted within population-based cancer registries are particularly suitable for the demonstration of associations between various types of cancer because observed and expected numbers of cancer cases derive from the same population. An example is provided by the tabulation of multiple primary cancers in Connecticut and Denmark, where more than 700 000 patients were studied (Boice et al., 1985). This study confirmed the constellation of multiple cancers of the breast, corpus uteri, ovary and colon, which has been related to hormonal factors (e.g. nulliparity) and dietary habits (e.g. high fat intake). Cervical cancer does not belong to this group, but rather to that of smoking-related cancers such as cancer of the respiratory tract. It should also be noted that the risk of breast cancer is reduced subsequent to cervical cancer. The explanation may be that risk factors for one cancer tend to be protective for the other or that radiation treatment induces castration. Data from the international cervical cancer study supports the latter hypothesis.

To elucidate further any possible hormonal factors involved in the etiology of cancers of the breast, ovary and corpus uteri, it is necessary to obtain detailed information on exogenous as well as endogenous sources of hormones, e.g. from medical records. This, combined with the relative scarcity of cases, makes the case-control design attractive.

The advantage of studying hormones used in the treatment of these cancers is that the dosage and duration of use are recorded very accurately. Doses may also be higher than those used for other purposes, which facilitates the detection of an increased risk. There are, however, several disadvantages. Most studies have to be carried out retrospectively over prolonged periods of time during which treatment modalities may change and drugs become obsolete. Hormonal treatments often start when metastases are discovered, and survival is consequently poor. This reduces the duration of use and the time necessary for a second cancer to develop. Finally, since both cases and controls have a high risk profile in terms of particular factors a certain degree of overmatching may occur. An example is provided by Ewertz et al. (1984).

REFERENCES

Boice, J.D., Storm, H.H., Curtis, R.E., Jensen, O.M., Kleinerman, R.A., Jensen, H.S., Flannery, J.T. & Fraumeni, J.F., eds (1985) Multiple Primary Cancers in Connecticut and Denmark. Natl. Cancer Inst. Monogr., 68

Ewertz, M., Machado, S.G., Boice, J.D. & Jensen, O.M. (1984) Endometrial cancer following treatment for breast cancer: A case-control study in Denmark. Br. J. Cancer, 50, 687-692

www.ingramcontent.com/pod-product-compliance
Ingram Content Group UK Ltd.
Pitfield, Milton Keynes, MK11 3LW, UK
UKHW051524180426
11947UKWH00018B/1563